A Guide to Massage Therapy

(Including Water Therapy)

Published by :
Lotus Press Publishers & Distributors

A Guide to Massage Therapy
(Including Water Therapy)

Dr. Rajeev Sharma
M.D., D.Lit.

Lotus PRESS

4735/22, Prakash Deep Building
Ansari Road, Darya Ganj,
New Delhi - 110002

Lotus Press : Publishers & Distributors
Unit No. 220, 2nd Floor, 4735/22, Prakash Deep Building,
Ansari Road, Darya Ganj, New Delhi- 110002
Ph.: 41325510, 98118-38000
• E-mail : lotuspress1984@gmail.com
www.lotuspress.co.in

A Guide to Massage Therapy

ISBN: 81-8382-160-X

Printed & Published by : **Lotus Press Publishers & Distributors,** New Delhi-02

About The Author

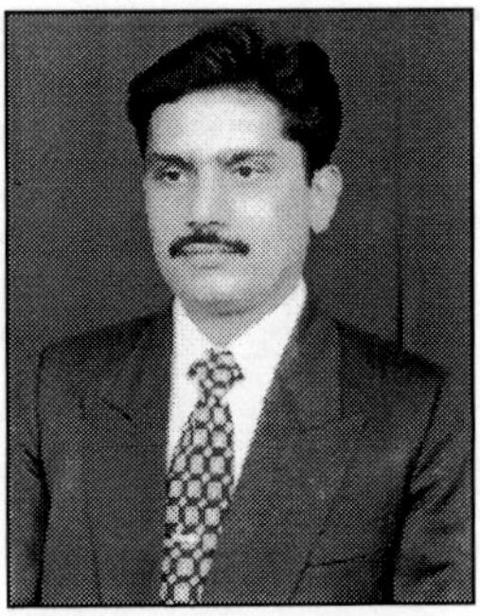

Dr. Rajeev Sharma

Dr. Rajeev Sharma is an eminent consultant of Homoeopathy, Yoga, Naturopathy and Alternative Medicine in India. He has written more than two hundred twenty five books (225) in Hindi and English and around one thousand articles which have been published in various newspapers and magazines. He is also an Editional Board Member of the prestigious Asian Homoeopathic Journal besides many other newspapers and magazines.

Dr. Rajeev Sharma has written books on ayurveda, homoe-opathy, yoga, naturopathy, accupressure, magnetotherapy, water-therapy, massage and aromatherapy etc., and on all major ailments.

Dr. Rajeev Sharma is Medical Advisor to Ralson Remedies (a homoeopathic manufacturer), and Dixit Pharmacy (Ayurvedic Manufacturer), Sr. Medical Officer U.P. Govt. He has received several prizes for his outstanding achievements. He has been awarded the *Best Author Prize in Hindi* by the Ministry of Health and Family Welfare, Government of India and *Sarjana Puraskar by U.P. Hindi Sansthan*, Lucknow. He has delivered talks on All India Radio and Total T.V. and lectures on Alternative Medicine in various Government and Non-government Organisations. He has written Advt. Scripts for the products of several companies.

He has established an institute through which you can get certificates by correspondence in Accupressure, Massage, Yoga, Water Therapy, Diet Therapy, Naturopathy, Colour Therapy and Reiki besides other paramedical courses.

He is providing literature on Personality Development and Life-Style Management.

Dr. Rajeev Sharma is also a social activist. He has worked a lot against Addiction and Prevention of AIDS. He has worked for population and pollution control and human rights and has received the World Human Rights Promotion Award. His name has been published in *LIMCA BOOK OF RECORDS,* 2005. He has developed a website too :- www.newkamasutra.com

Dr. Rajeev Sharma is National President of an NGO UTKRISHTA BHARAT (An All India Association of Socio-Cultural Religious and Sports Activities).

Preface

Massage is a relaxing technique which is accepted all over the world. Massage in India is prevalent since ancient times. Massage if done scientifically, is very effective and relaxes body thoroughly.

The word massage is derived from Greek Language, signifying to knead, to press. It consists basically of palpation, rubbing and kneading. Celsus, a Roman physician, at the beginning of Christian era advised that friction should be used several times a day in the sun and found that chronic pains in the head were relieved by rubbing the head itself and the paralysed limbs were strengthened by being rubbed.

To take bath after oil massage was a common custom in Turkey and Kerala. By simple massage one can keep his body ever young.

By massage, the whole body, the skin, the muscles, the veins, the arteries, the lymphatic's and the whole nervous system is benefitted.

This book provides the scientific techniques of massage, oil used in massage, essential oils (aroma's), beauty treatments, skincare; care of hands, foot etc.

Besides massage, there is a detailed information on water treatment. Water is not only essential for our body as a drink, it helps in treating various disorders also.

Hope, readers will be benefitted by this book.

Dr. Rajeev Sharma

Srijan—Aarogya Jyoti®
Palm—11/03, Shipra Sun City
Ghaziabad (U.P.)
Ph.: 0120-6460127
email: sharmarajeev108@rediffmail.com

Contents

1

Types of Massage

Basically there are seven types of massage and eigth one is combined action.

- Touching
- Tapping (Stroke)
- Friction
- Pressing (Rubbing by pressure)
- Vibrating
- Rolling
- Patting, and
- Combined action

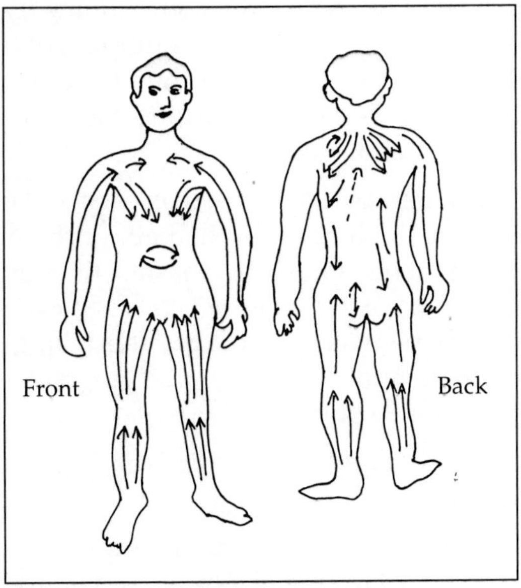

Scientific Massage

Touching: The organs of the patient are touched by giving pressure by fingers or by soft hands. This technique is useful for weak patients. Massage technique starts through it. By touching near the spine of the patient, he becomes energetic and his muscles are stimulated.

Tapping: In this technique muscles and tissues of the body are given strokes slowly. If the muscles ache, tapping therapy is essential. The technique of touching and tapping are changed according to the condition of the patient.

Friction: Hands or dry towel is used in this technique. One can do it himself. If the patient is stocked or has fainted due to cold, friction technique can be adopted. The head of the patient on the bed should be downwards and his feet and hands should be given vigorous friction. It would improve natural blood circulation in his body.

Pressing (Rubbing by pressure): Discomfort created by standing in train or bus for a long period or by working till late or the troubles created by mental tension, rubbing by pressure technique relieves much. By pressing the muscles of thighs and calf muscles and near the spine, the muscles are toned and nerves are stimulated. For example, forehead is pressed by hands to get relief from headache.

Vibrating: This therapy can be used on each and every part of the body. It gives much relief in the pain of the muscles of the back and headache. One can master this therapy by constant practice. If done by balanced hands, it gives relief at once. It makes the patient sleep at once. After taking enema in the lower abdomen and intestines, this therapy helps in expelling toxic substance out of the body.

Rolling: Keep right hand over the limb and left hand under it. Roll both the hands in opposite direction, *i.e.* up and down.

Patting: The best example of this therapy is patting the back of the child in her lap to make him sleep. Patting should be done in a very slow process.

Combined Actions: The massage therapist should be well acquainted and well practised with all the above techniques of massage. Only one technique of massage is neither sufficient for the body nor upto the liking of the patient While massaging the body, the therapist should adopt all the techniques of vibration, friction and pressure by rubbing. Combined techniques of massage give it perfection.

INSTRUCTIONS FOR MASSAGE THERAPIST

The massage therapist should always follow the directions given below:

- The massage therapist should be of pure mind and body. He should massage with the feeling of service.
- The effects of massage are not only on body but on mind also. A person can inculcate his good or bad feelings in the other person by touching. The masseur should be having sympathetic attitude.
- If he is engrossed in good thinking, or prayers to God, he is blessed with supernatural powers and he massages the patient more attentively.
- The person doing the massage should be clean and active. He should wear least clothes so that he may attentively massage the patient without wasting his time and attention in caring his clothes.
- Hands, feet and hair have their inclination towards fingers and the massage is done towards the just opposite side. In such a situation, oil for massage should be used in more quantity so that the hair might not break. If the hair are broken, small eruptions occur on that place, which ache much.
- The masseur sweats much while doing the massage. He should keep a small towel to wipe the sweat so that it may not fall upon the patient.
- The movements of hands at the time of massage should be towards heart. For example, if you have to massage

legs, start with the massage of the fingers of the feet and then ankles, knees and thighs. Blood circulation with the heart beat reaches upto small cells of the organs of the body through small nerves divided from the large artery. Blood circulation in artery gets push through heart.

- Physical and mental exhaustion cause slowness in blood circulation in the arteries and veins and it can be cured by massage.
- The aim of the masage should be to maintain blood circulation without causing extra labour to heart.
- One should try to keep his body and the organs concerned stable at the time of the massage.
- One should take sufficient oil on his palm before starting massage.

■

2

Aroma-Massage Principles—Do's and Dont's

Remember how as a child if you bumped your head (or anywhere else) a wise adult would kindly rub it better? Or that if any part of your body aches now it's instinctive to put your hand there?

Very simply, this how massage works. Touch is both healing and comforting and, what's more, we can all enjoy the pleasures of it—both giving and receiving. Massage is beneficial to us in several different ways:

- ☞ Improves blood circulation
- ☞ Calms the nervous system
- ☞ Stimulates skin function
- ☞ Improves muscle tone
- ☞ Eases aches and pains in muscles and joints

And it feels marvellous!

THE BASIC PRINCIPLES OF MASSAGE

In basic terms massage is a way of stroking the body, with variations in the length and depth of strokes. However, you should always direct firm strokes towards the heart, as this will be beneficial to the circulation.

Long flowing massage strokes with little pressure on the body are the most soothing and relaxing. This type of movement is called effleurage. It is done with the whole hand using gentle, even pressure and is often used to start and finish a massage.

Patting or tapping the skin with your fingers quickly and slowly is stimulating and helps to increase blood flow. This is called tapotement: It is usually done on small areas such as the forehead, cheeks and neck.

Petrissage involves squeezing and releasing a muscle or part of a muscle group. A good example of this kind of movement is kneading dough. It is mostly done with both hands, particularly on the thighs and buttocks. Petrissage helps strengthen muscle fibre, remove waste products and ease fatigue.

There's another type of massage movement called friction which creates just that. It involves rubbing the hands backwards and forwards across an area and is very warming and stimulating to the tissues. Rubbing our hands quickly together on a freezing winter day is a good example of how friction can work.

A professional aromatherapist uses mainly effleurage and works on pressure points with some frictions and petrissage, but there is no reason why you can't vary the movement if you decide you would like to try giving a simple massage.

You don't need to be an expert to give a soothing massage to family or friends. Once you've learned a few basic movements you'll probably be in demand.

Dos and Dont's

Massage is a gentle healing art suitable for everyone from babies to the very elderly. However, there are certain times or conditions when it should be avoided (for example, when the person has just eaten a heavy meal). Often, this just means leaving out a body area but use your common sense and if unsure leave well done.

Do not massage

- ☞ Any infected area.
- ☞ A person who is feverish or has a raised temperature.

- ☞ Over an area where varicose veins are present.
- ☞ Over any unusual swelling or inflammation.
- ☞ Bruised or broken skin.

Before massaging do

- ☞ Check with the person about to be massaged whether any of the above apply.
- ☞ Make sure the room is warm enough.
- ☞ Warm your hands before massaging—cold hands are a real shock. Not a good way to begin!

■

3

Creating the Right Atmosphere

Wouldn't it be wonderful to be massaged in a tropical country, with the warm sun beating down, soft sounds of the sea in the background and the sweet scents of flowers occasionally wafting over you?

Well, perhaps it's rather a far-fetched dream but it is still possible to create a lovely, relaxing atmosphere at home, especially with the help of aromatherapy oils. I think the most important consideration is that the room, or area, you use to give a massage is really warm. Believe me, there's nothing more shivering and covered with goose pimples. Remember that while a person is lying still he or she generates less body heat: you know how difficult it is to get off to sleep if you feel really cold in bed.

It's a good idea to have a blanket, or large towel, so you can cover the parts of the body you are not working on. Also, it feels good to be wrapped up while being massaged. If you like, you can even wrap a hot water bottle in a towel and pop it under your patient's feet for a really luxurious treat.

Harsh, bright lights are unpleasant when being massaged. Obviously, until you feel confident in what you are doing you'll need a reasonalbe amount of light, just to see clearly as you go. A table lamp is sufficient for this: it gives a softer, gentler light than overhead lighting. Once you feel happy about your massage movements you can work by candlelight. The soft flickering of the flames has a soothing, hypnotic effect which is really relaxing.

Try to keep noise to the minimum, and close the curtains or blinds. This helps to cut out traffic noise. If you think you may be disturbed, unplug the telephone. It's now possible to buy some really interesting tapes to play in the background. Sounds of the sea, tinkling bells, birdsong and running water all combined with gentle, lulling music can take you off into a dreamlike state.

Part of the benefits of aromatherapy massage is the feeling of getting away from stressful day-to-day living, so music can be a great help in creating a relaxing atmosphere. This is a very personal thing and you'll find out for yourself which sounds are most relaxing for you. I find playing the tapes helps me to relax more while I am giving a massage, too, even when the day has been hectic and I am feeling less than calm.

Aromatherapy oils are marvellous for creating different atmospheres in the home and are much more authentic than using chemical copies or perfume sprays. Smells seem to strongly imprint themselves on our memories, and a certain aroma can evoke all sorts of feelings from the past. For example, the smell of warm spices, such a cinnamon and cloves, always reminds me of Christmasses spent at my grandparents'. And the sweet, sickly scent of benzoin reminds me of the day my little sister drank half a bottle of friar's balsam thinking it was some sort of chocolate drink!

There are several ways of scenting your home with essential oils. The simplest is probably to add a few drops of your chosen oil to a small bowl of water and then stand it over a radiator. The essentail oil floats on the water and gradually evaporates into the air, aided by the heat.

A more sophisticated method is to use an oil burner or vaporizer. These come in many different designs, but with the oil burners there is no need to use any water. You just put a few drops of essential oil into the top of the burner, then light a night light underneath. Vaporizers usually have a deeper dish into which you add water, followed by your favourite essential oil. However, whether you use an oil burner or a vaporizer, do be careful not to let it burn dry!

Used in this way to oils can become mood enhancers. They can remove stale smells or even help with conditions such as headaches, colds or insomnia.

Another way to perfume a room is to make your own pot-pourri. Gather flowers and herbs from your garden and hang them up in bundles to dry. (The airing cupboard is the ideal place for this.) Once dried, crumble them together, keeping some of the smaller flower heads intact. Now you are ready to perfume your pot-pourri with the essential oils of your choice. Generally, I find it better to use single essences rather than a blend.

Here are few suggestions:

Fresh and light Lemon, coriander, vetivert and melissa.

Warm and spicy Benzoin, cinnamon, clove and patchouli.

Sweet and flowery Lavender, neroli, ylang-ylang sandalwood.

You can also boost a tired pot-pourri by using aromatherapy oils in the same way.

Another way to perfume a room is with a light bulb ring. This is either a ceramic or metal ring which sits on a light bulb. Once the ring is in place all you do is pour in a few drops of essential oil. The fragrance is more effective when the light is turned on as the heat increases the oil's evaporation.

Now you have a few ideas on how to create a warm, relaxing atmosphere for aromatherapy massage we can look at the massage techniques in more detail. As I mentioned before, everyone can learn to give a simple massage; you'll be surprised at how enjoyable it can be.

■

4

Oils and Herbs for Different Diseases

Oils and herbs which are available at home are effective for preparing massage oil and they cure several diseases. They cost very little when compared to commercial preparations. They are as follows:

1. Mustard oil,
2. Til oil,
3. Camphor oil,
4. Eucalyptus oil,
5. Almond oil,
6. Olive oil,
7. Coconut oil,
8. Castor oil, and
9. Herbs available in kitchen.

DISEASES CONCERNED WITH RESPIRATION

1. Add camphor powder to coconut oil and heat it slightly. It gives relief in common cold, rattling phelgm in the chest and cough.
2. It should be rubbed on the nose for common cold. It should be rubbed on the throat for throat cough and on chest for chest cough.
3. If the nose is blocked, massage with two or three drops of mustard oil on the nose.

Asthma, Bronchitis

Take two spoons of garlic juice and mix it in half a cup of til oil. Heat the oil till the juice evaporates. Remove it from fire.

Cool and store it in a bottle. Heat it before use and massage on the chest.

Digestive Problems

Pain in Stomach and Constipation.

Heat castor oil slightly and massage it around and above the navel. It will give relief in stomach cramps and pain and remove constipation.

Flaulence and Fullness

Add a pinch of Asafoetida powder in til oil or mustard oil. Heat it slightly and rub on the abdomen.

Skin Diseases

Add dry curry leaves to coconut oil and keep it in the sun for 15 days. Massage this oil on the skin two hours before bath. This cures and prevents any type of itching and eruption. It gives bright glow to the skin and makes it healthy.

Arthritis and Rheumatism

1. If the pain is mild and tolerable, massage mustard oil on the affected part.
2. Powder Ajwain and extract oil from it. Massage the painful joints with oil.
3. Add 10 to 15 cloves to 4 table spoons of til oil and heat. When the garlic becomes black, remove it from fire and add one spoon camphor powder. Rub this oil three to four times a day.
4. If the pain is chronic with inflammation, the herbal oil should be prepared as following:
   - *i.* 200 gm til oil
   - *ii.* 1 spoon of Ajwain
   - *iii.* 1 spoon of cloves
   - *iv.* 8 garlic pieces. Peel them and crush them.
   - *v.* 2 spoons mustard seeds.

Heat oil and add mustard seeds to splutter. Powder Ajwain and cloves. Add all these ingredients to the oil and stir well. The garlic should turn black. Remove it from fire, cool and store in a bottle. Rub this oil on the affected joints.

Spinal Massage

- ☞ Massage must not be given on the bones of spine directly but two inches from the centre. Massage on either side of spine assists in curing the organs of the front side of the body.
- ☞ Divide the back into upper and lower divisions. Massage on either side of the spine on the upper division to treat diseases of lungs, heart, stomach, liver and other digestive organs. Massage either side of spine on the lower division to cure the diseases of the kidneys, intestines, urinary and menstrual problems.

MUSTARD OIL AND ITS BENEFICIAL PROPERTIES

Mustard oil is used frequently in our country India. It is often used in cooking food. Massage with mustard oil is most prevalent in India. Use of pure yellow mustard oil is considered the best. Mustard oil contains various properties which are effective in curing diseases.

Mustard oil is used in our daily life in the following ways:

1. Its massage in the body gives energy and strength. The bones of the body become strong.
2. Warm the mustard oil with garlic. When garlic becomes black, remove it from the fire, cool it and massage it on the body of a child. This prescription has a curative effect.
3. Mix the powdered salt with the mustard oil. Rub it on the teeth. It cleanses the teeth and gives relief in pain. Some persons use it daily to cleanse the teeth.
4. If hand and feet are aching, massage with mustard oil.

5. Massage with mustard oil on head relieves headache.
6. If there is dirt and filth in the ear and it is aching, pour some drops of lukewarm mustard oil. It will relieve the pain soon.
7. If the hand and feet are rough and dry, massage lightly with mustard oil. Massage with mustard oil cures dryness and the skin becomes soft.
8. If you are too tired, warm the mustard oil with garlic and massage the soles with it, you will be relaxed beyond expectation.
9. The fingers of the feet become tender by working continuously in water. Regular massage of them with mustard oil cures them.
10. After massage, one should take sunbath for sometime in winter season. It gives glow to the skin and the bones become strong. One should take bath after half an hour of sunbath.

■

5

Carrier Oils

Carrier oils or base oils are vegetable, nut or seed oils. Many of these carrier oils also have therapeutic properties. Vegetable oils are extracted from the seeds of the plants. Vegetable oils contain a good amount of proteins nutrients and energy. They enable the body to produce heat and lubrication.

The essential oils are very highly concentrated and cannot be used directly on the skin. The essential oils are hence diluted with a base or carrier oil so that they can be massaged or rubbed into the skin in the correct proportion.

Almond Oil (Sweet)

Colour : Very pale yellow

Extracted : from the kernel

Contains : glycosides, minerals, vitamins and proteins

Uses : good for skin, helps relieve itching, soreness, dryness and inflammation

Base oil : Can be used as a base without dilution

Apricot kernel Oil

Colour : pale yellow

Extracted : from the kernel

Contains : minerals, vitamins

Uses : all types of skin particularly for prematured aged, sensitive, inflammed and dry skin

Base oil : can be used as a base without dilution

Avocado Pear Oil

Colour : dark green

Extracted : from the fruit

Contains : vitamins, proteins, lecithin and fatty acids

Uses : all types of skin especially dry and dehydrated skin, eczema

Base oil : to be used as an addition to a base oil in 10 percent dilution

Carrot Oil

Colour : Orange

Contains : vitamins, minerals, and beta-carotene

Uses : premature aging, itching, dryness, psoriasis and eczema
Very rejuvenating by itself and reduces scarring

Base oil : to be used as an addition to a base oil in 10 percent dilution
Do not use undiluted directly on the skin

Corn Oil

Colour : Pale Yellow

Contains : minerals, vitamins and protein

Uses : Soothing for all types of skin

Base oil : can be used as a base oil

Evening Primrose Oil

Colour : Pale Yellow

Contains : vitamins, minerals, and gamma linolenic acid

Uses : during Pre menstrual tension, multiple sclerosis, menopause related tensions, heart diseases. Excerllent while treating eczema and psoriasis. Helps prevent premature aging of skin

Base oil : use in 10 percent dilution.

Grapeseed Oil

Colour : nearly colourless or pale green

Contains : vitamins, minerals, and protein

Uses : for all types of skin

Base oil : can be used as base oil without dilution

Hazelnut Oil

Colour : Yellow

Extracted : from the kernel

Contains : vitamins, minerals, and protein

Uses : for all types of skin. It has a slight astringent action

Base oil : use with 10 percent dilution

Peanut Oil

Colour : Pale Yellow

Contains : vitamins, minerals, and protein

Uses : for all types of skin

Base oil : can be used as base oil without dilution

Safflower Oil

Colour : Pale Yellow

Contains : vitamins, minerals, and protein

Uses : for all types of skin

Base oil : can be used as base oil without dilution

Sesame Oil

Colour : Dark Yellow

Contains : vitamins, minerals, protein, lecithin and amino acids

Uses : rheumatism, arthritis, psoriasis, eczema. Useful for all types of skin

Base oil : use in 10 percent dilution

Soya bean Oil

Colour	:	Pale Yellow
Contains	:	vitamins, minerals, and protein
Uses	:	for all types of skin
Base oil	:	can be used as base oil without dilution

Sunflower Oil

Colour	:	Pale Yellow
Contains	:	vitamins, minerals, and protein
Uses	:	for all types of skin
Base oil	:	can be used as base oil without dilution.

■

6

Chief Essential Oils and Their Benefits

These essentials oils are very useful, if used with carrier oils.

Amrette Seed

Botanical name	:	Abelmoschus Moschatus
Plant part	:	Seeds
Properties	:	Warmth-giving, relaxing, stimulating, calming
Quantity	:	2-3 drops
Application	:	Helpful in relieving anxiety, fatigue, depression or other stress-related conditions, muscular aches, pains, cramps and poor circulation. Is an aphrodisiac. Excellent to freshen up tired and hurting feet.
Precaution	:	Use in low dosage. Avoid very frequent massages or baths.

Aniseed

Botanical name	:	Pimpenella Anisum
Plant part	:	Seed pod
Properties	:	Warming, stimulating
Quantity	:	3-5 drops
Application	:	Helpful in treating coughs, bronchitis and catarrh.

Angelica

Botanical name	:	Angelica Archangelica
Plant part	:	Root, seed, fruit
Properties	:	Expectorant, digestive stimulant, relaxing
Quantity	:	2-3 drops
Application	:	Useful for colds, coughs, flu, muscular pains and aches, rheumatism. Helps in digestion. Also useful in healing smoker's cough.
Precaution	:	Avoid during pregnancy. Can cause photosensitivity so avoid exposure to sun after use.

Basil

Botanical name	:	Ocimum Basilicum
Plant part	:	Leaves
Properties	:	Uplifting, refreshing
Quantity	:	2-3 drops
Application	:	Good for students and executives. Helps in relieving nervous tension, stress, mild anxiety, nausea, indigestion, flatulence, loss of appetite, temporarily relieves cough, sinusitis, cold, fever, bronchitis, earaches, eases muscular pains, spasm, rheumatic and arthritic pains. It also acts as an insect repellent.
Precaution	:	Avoid during pregnancy.

Bergamot

Botanical name	:	Citrus Aurantium
Plant part	:	Peel of the fruit
Properties	:	Calming, refreshing, rejuvenating
Quantity	:	3-5 drops

Application : Heals wounds and relieves ulcers, treats eczema, psoriasis (stress related) and PMT (pre Menstrual Tension). Works as an appetiser. Beneficial in treating oily skin problems. Relieves respiratory infections viz bronchitis, sore throat and tonsilitis, colic, flatulence and indigestion. Beneficial in treating anxiety, depression, mental and psychological disturbances. Acts as an antiseptic for urinary tract problem, cystitis. Effective in treating cold sores, chicken pox and shingles.

Precaution : Avoid using on sensitive skin as it can cause irritation. Avoid exposure to sun as it can increase skin's photosensitivity.

Black Pepper

Botanical name : Piper Nigrum

Plant part : Berry

Properties : Warming, strenthening

Quantity : 2-3 drops

Application : Helps in relieving muscular aches, pains, stiffness, fatigue. Useful in relieving physical and emotional problems. Gives temporary relief from arthritis, fibrosis, cold, flu, indigestion, respiratory infections, chills, catarrh. Helps in curing colic, flatulence, indigestion, heart burn and loss of appetite. Helps to maintain peripheral circulation, eases chilblains and tones muscles. Increases concentration and alertness.

Precaution : Use in moderation.

Camphor

Botanical name : Cinnamomum Camphora

Plant part : Wood
Properties : Relieving
Quantity : 2-3 drops
Application : Helps in treating coughs, colds, fevers, rheumatism, arthritis constipation, insomnia, sprains, dep-ression, acne and inflammed skin.
Precaution : Use in moderation.

Cardamom

Botanical name : Elettaria cardomumum
Plant part : Seeds
Properties : Warming
Quantity : 2-3 drops
Application : Helps in relieving nausea, coughs, headaches, aches, digestion and it is a tonic
Precaution : Use in moderation.

Chamomile

Botanical name : Matricaria Chamomilia
Plant part : Flowers
Properties : Soothes
Quantity : 3-5 drops
Application : Eases anxiety, anger and fear, helpful in treating insomnia, used for colitis, gastritis, diarrhoea, urinary tract infection, meno-pause and menstrual related problems. Relieves stress, depression and irritability related to PMT. Helps to relieve muscular pains, inflammation of arthritic joints and swollen joints. It is used in treating skin problems viz. psoriasis, dermatitis and eczema. Mild on children facing teething problem and earache. Soothes burns, blisters, inflammed wounds, broken

		capillaries. It can be used to lighten fair hair.
Precaution	:	Avoid during pregnancy.

Clove Bud

Botanical name	:	Syzygium Aromaticum
Plant part	:	Buds
Properties	:	Warming and soothing
Quantity	:	1-2 drops
Application	:	Relieves aches and pains (joints). Rheumatoid sprains, asthma, colds, flu, colic, dyspepsia, nausea, diarrhoea, toothache, ulcers, wounds, bronchitis, nervous tension, depression and stress. It is used as an effective antiseptic, and analgesic anti-bacterial. Useful as mosquito repellent and in fighting acne. Helps relieve athlete's foot and cuts.
Precaution	:	Use in low moderation. Avoid during pregnancy.

Cypress

Botanical name	:	Cupressus Sempervirens
Plant part	:	Needles, twigs
Properties	:	Refreshing, calming and strengthening
Quantity	:	2 drops
Application	:	An astringent to circulation, haemorhoids, varicose veins, cellulite; brings down external bleeding and excessive perspiration and heavy menstrual flow; useful in asthma, bronchitis, dry cough, cold and flu. Helps to heal swollen breasts.
Precaution	:	Avoid during pregnancy.

Clary Sage

Botanical name	:	Salvia Sclarea
Plant part	:	Flowering tops
Properties	:	Euphoric, sensual, warming and relaxing
Quantity	:	2-5 drops
Application	:	Useful in dealing with anxiety, stress, tension and migraine, menstrual cramps and pains, PMT, muscular tension, excessive perspiration. Being warming and relaxing nourishes conversation. Brings down high blood pressure and excessive sebum. Reduces post natal depression and eases child birth by encouraging labour. Immune system gets strengthened. Eases asthma.
Precaution	:	Can cause drowsiness, avoid when under alcoholic effect. Avoid during pregnancy and also if one suffers from epilepsy.

Eucalyptus

Botanical name	:	Eucalptus Globulus
Plant part	:	Leaves, twigs
Properties	:	Cooling and clearing
Quantity	:	2-3 drops
Application	:	Clears stuffed nose and head. Acts as a decongestant; cures fever, cold. Relieves stress, fatigue, muscular pains, sprains, aches, rheumatism, headaches, sinusitis and mild respiratory infections. It is anti-inflammatory. Quite useful in treating wounds, burns, boils, abscesses, blisters, cold sore, shingles, blemishes, insect bites, anti-bacterial and is an insect repellent too.

Precaution : Can irritate skin. Keep away from children.

Fennel

Botanical name : Foeniculum Vulgare

Plant part : Seeds

Properties : Calming

Quantity : 2-3 drops

Application : Useful in easing colic, constipation and digestion problems, fluid retention, cellulite, menstrual pain, PMT, menopause, nausea, flatulence and loss of appetite. Helps in fighting hangovers, increases flow of breast milk and relieves bronchitis. Cures kidney stones and relieves intestinal spasm. Has a mild diuretic and laxative effect.

Precaution : Avoid during pregnancy.

Frankincense

Botanical name : Olibanum Boswellia Carterii

Plant part : Gum resin

Properties : Fortifying, soothing

Quantity : 3-5 drops

Application : Helps in meditation; slows and deepens breathing. Fortifies emotionally against nightmares, fear and grief. Balances and opens Crown chakra. It helps in healing ulcers and infected wounds. Treats dry, wrinkled, inflamed skin. It also cures coughs, laryngitis, asthma, catarrh and bronchitis. It reduces scar and promotes healing. Aids in maintaining supple skin by toning it.

Geranium

Botanical name : Pelargonium Graveolens
Plant part : Leaves, stalk, flower
Properties : Calming, balancing, relaxing, refreshing
Quantity : 5-7 drops
Application : Helps to deal with nervous tension, anxiety, mood swings, depression, menopause problems, hot flushes, post natal depression, PMT, irregular menstruation. Treats swollen and painful breasts, fluid retention problems, emotional outbursts, irritability, throat infections. It cures colds, flu, neuralgia, sciatica, acne, bruises, burns, cuts, eczema, burns, cuts, dermatitis, eczema, mature skin and mouth ulcers. Normalises skin imbalances. Works as insect repellant, harmonises and calms. It also acts as an astringent and cleanser.

Ginger

Botanical name : Zingiber Officinale
Plant part : Root
Properties : Warming, stimulating
Quantity : 2 drops
Application : Relieves colic, cramp, flatulence, nausea, travel sickness and indigestion. Cures migraine, coughs, congestion, common cold, catarrh, influenza, sore throat, sinusitis, arthritic pains, rheumatism, muscular aches, sprains and strains. Helps in blood circulation and aids memory. Heals bones and brings down temperature in fever also. Relieves morning sickness (if inhaled) in pregnancy and hangovers. Stimulates

		circulation, relaxes blood vessels and can also help ease angina.
Precaution	:	Use in low moderation. May irritate sensitive skin.

Juniper Berry

Botanical name	:	Juniperus Communis
Plant part	:	Berries
Properties	:	Uplifting, refreshing, relaxing
Quantity	:	2-3 drops
Application	:	Used to relive stress, anxiety, pains of joints and rheumatic pain. Heals bruises, cramps, acne, colic, coughs, arthritis, menstrual pain, less menstrual flow, swollen and painful breasts (pre-menstrual). Deals with fluid retention, cellulite, obesity, poor circulation, haemorrohoids, loss of appetite. Tones the skin.
Precaution	:	Avoid during pregnancy and if suffering from high blood pressure. Can irritate the kidneys if used in excess.

Lavender

Botanical name	:	Lavandula Angustifolia
Plant part	:	Flowers
Properties	:	Harmonising, soothing, balancing, refreshing, relaxing, calming
Quantity	:	5-10 drops
Application	:	Aids in relieving irritability (in adults and children as well), anxiety, stress. Relieves muscular aches and pains, bites and stings. Cures colds, flu, insomnia, headach, minor burns and scalds. It is anti-fungal and anti-bacterial so it is very useful in treating

		wounds. It can be used directly to relieve pain of minor burns and scalds. It balances and harmonises the body.
Precaution	:	Avoid during early pregnancy.

Lemon

Botanical name	:	Citrus Limon
Plant part	:	Peel of fruit
Properties	:	Rejuvenating, enlivening, cooling, uplifting
Quantity	:	3-6 drops
Application	:	Helps in healing bronchial problems, colds, flu, fever, sore throat, mouth ulcers, hormonal headaches, poor circulation, high blood pressure, wounds, stress, nervous tension and counteracts acidity. Aids in clearing freckels and to rid warts. Useful for students and executives. Helps in stopping hot flushes in menopause. It has an enliving and refreshing aroma and is an effective insect repellent too.
Precaution	:	Causes photo-sensitivity on sensitive skin. Avoid using when going out in sun as it may irritate sensitive skin.

Lemongrass

Botanical name	:	Cymbogen Citratus
Plant part	:	Grass
Properties	:	Tranquilizing, soothing calming, refreshing
Quantity	:	1-3 drops
Application	:	Helps in relieving shock, grief, trauma, depression and stress. Helps to fight lethargy, irritability during PMT and menopause, insomnia, excitability in children, chronic diarrhoea triggered due to emotional reasons. Improves skin

elasticity, thread veins, stretch marks and scars. It gives relief from headaches, sore throat and mild respiratory problems. Helps in opening the skin pores, treating oily skin, curing acne and relieves indigestion.

Precaution : Avoid during pregnancy. It can also irritate skin.

Marjoram

Botanical name : Origanum Marjorana

Plant part : Flowers, leaves

Properties : Calming, warming

Quantity : 3-5 drops

Application : Relieves anxiety, stress, high blood pressure, arthritis, rheumatism, swollen joints, asthma, colds, flu, sinusitis. Cures migraines, stomach and menstrual cramps, indigestion, constipation and flatulence. Calming to the nervous system. Reduces sexual urges, heals bruises.

Precaution : Use in moderation. Avoid during pregnancy.

Neroli

Botanical name : Citus Aurantium

Plant part : Petals

Properties : Calming, soothing, refreshing

Quantity : 1-3 drops

Application : Relieves mental lethargy, headaches, irritability caused due to menopause and PMT. It cures chronic diarrhoea due to emotional state and thread veins. Cures dryness, improves elasticity, sensitivity of skin and is also kind on mature skin.

Calms excitable and restless children when used in baths before going to bed. Helps during shocks, trauma, grief and stress. Highly calming to those suffering from anxiety and fears. Helps lighten stretch marks and scars. Soothes palpitation, stress related problems and depression. Helps during pregnancy and labour.

Orange (Sweet)

Botanical name	:	Citrus Aurantium
Plant part	:	Peel
Properties	:	Calming, refreshing
Quantity	:	2-3 drops
Application	:	Effective in healing mouth ulcers, treats nervous tension, stress and anxiety. Gives relief from bronchial coughs, colds, flu and insomnia. Eases constipation and diarrhoea. It is very gentle on children brings down the fever.
Precaution	:	May increase skin photo-sensitivity. Avoid use before going out in the sun.

Palmarosa

Botanical name	:	Cymbopogon Martinii
Plant part	:	Grass
Properties	:	Clarifying, uplifting calming, refreshing
Quantity	:	4-5 drops
Application	:	Stimulates cell regeneration, circulation, appetite. It maintains a supple skin, removes scars, helpful in treating acne, dermatitis balances sebum production, relieves indigestion, colds, flu, viruses and reduces fever.

Peppermint

Botanical name : Mentha piperita

Plant part : Leaves

Properties : Cooling, invigorating comforting, refreshing, calming

Quantity : 1-3 drops

Application : A decongestant which gives relief from asthma, colds, flu, fever, headaches, toothaches, sinusitis, nausea, travel sickness, stomach upsets and indigestion, hangover. Cools skin inflammation, burns and sunburns as it is very refreshing skin oil. Repels mosquitoes, mice and rats.

Precaution : Use in moderation as it can irritate sensitive skin. Avoid during early pregnancy.

Patchouli

Botanical name : Pogostemon Cabin

Plant part : Leaves

Properties : Warming, exotic, calming, relaxing, enlivening

Quantity : 2-4 drops

Application : Exotic aroma often used in perfumery. Emotionally enlivening, excites the senses. Helps in relieving anxiety, stress, and depression. Helps to heal chapped rough skin, wounds and sores. Being anti-inflammatory it helps cool inflammed skin. Effective in treating dandruff, scars. It is an anti-septic, astringent, anti-bacterial and insect repellent.

Precaution : Use in moderation as excess dose can cause sedation.

Petitgrain

Botanical name	:	Citrus Aurantium var Amara
Plant part	:	Leaves
Properties	:	Clarifying, soothing, uplifting
Quantity	:	4-5 drops
Application	:	Useful to relieve mental strain, restlessness, anxiety, tension, stress, flatulence, dyspepsia and constipation. Helps in stimulating digestion and poor memory. Brings down acne. Reduces excessive perspiration, treats greasy skin and hair. Helps to build up resistance to illness.

Pine

Botanical name	:	Pinus Sylvestris
Plant part	:	Needles
Properties	:	Invigorating, refreshing
Quantity	:	1-3 drops
Application	:	Relieves muscular aches, pains, Arthritis, rheumatism, poor circulation, asthma, bronchitis, coughs, catarrh, sinusitis, sore throats, colds, flu, nervous exhaustion, stress, fatigue, neuralgia, sciatica, poor concentration. Heals cuts and abrasions, excessive perspiration. It is also an effective insect repellent.

Rose

Botanical name	:	Rose Centifoda damascena
Plant part	:	Leaves and flowers
Properties	:	Exciting, balancing
Quantity	:	1-4 drops
Application	:	Helps to ease depression, frigidity, nervous tension, headache and insomnia.

Relieves asthma, shock, palpitations, poor circulation, dry coughs, nausea. Treats PMT, irregular or heavy menstruation, menstural pain, impotence, irritability. Hormonally balancing. Useful also for dry, chapped, aging skin and eczema.

Rosemary

Botanical name	:	Rosemarinus officinalis
Plant part	:	Leaves and flowers
Properties	:	Reviving, invogorating, focusing, refreshing
Quantity	:	2-4 drops
Application	:	Useful tonic for hair as it keeps dandruff at day, clears lice, adds lustre to the hair. Useful in relieving stress, mental fatigue, anxiety, muscular aches and pains, rheumatism, arthritis, gout, sinusitis, migraine colds, flu, asthma, respiratory problem, poor circulation, fluid retention, cellulite, menstrual cramps, scanty flow during menstruation. Helps aid better concentration and clarity while studying.
Precaution	:	Avoid during pregnancy, if suffering from blood pressure or epilepsy.

Sandalwood

Botanical name	:	Santalum Album
Plant part	:	Wood
Properties	:	Strengthening, sedating, calming, relaxing
Quantity	:	2-5 drops
Application	:	Helps to relieve nervous tension, depression, stress, anxiety, irritability, insomnia, dry coughs, sore throat, bronchitis, nausea, travel sickness. Heals inflamed, cracked,

dry, chapped, mature, aging skin, acne, blemishes and scars. Acts as a deodoriser in case of excessive perspiration. Excites the senses. It is an effective insect repellent.

Tarragon

Botanical name	:	Artemisia Dracunculus
Plant part	:	Leaves
Properties	:	Calming
Quantity	:	2-3 drops
Application	:	Useful to relieving stomach disorders, nervousness leading to butterflies or knots in the stomach, indigestion, flatulence, PMT, cramps, constipation. It is anti-spasmodic, antiseptic and slightly diuretic.
Precaution	:	Avoid during pregnancy. Use in moderation.

Tea tree

Botanical name	:	Melaleuca Alternifolia
Plant part	:	Leaves, twigs
Properties	:	Soothing
Quantity	:	2-5 drops
Application	:	Helpful in healing fungal and yeast infections, colds, influenza, cold sores, warts, burns, shock, bacterial and viral infections, stings, herpes, nappy rash and hysteria.

Thyme (White)

Botanical name	:	Thymus Vulgaris
Plant part	:	Leaves, flowers
Properties	:	Stimulating, invigorating
Quantity	:	2 drops
Application	:	Helpful in relieving tension, fatigue, anxiety, headaches, skin irritations,

		coughs, colds, rheumatic aches and pains. Useful insect repellent. It is a very good stimulant and expectorant.
Precaution	:	Avoid during pregnancy. Use in moderation.

Vetiver

Botanical name	:	Vetiveria Zizanoides
Plant part	:	Roots
Properties	:	Calming, balancing, grounding
Quantity	:	1-3 drops
Application	:	Helpful in relieving nervous tension, stress, muscular aches, pains, sprains, stiffness, arthritis, rheumatism, palpitation, congestion. Heals acne, blemishes, cuts and wound.

Ylang Ylang

Botanical name	:	Cananga Odorate
Plant part	:	Flowers
Properties	:	Balancing, relaxing
Quantity	:	2-3 drops
Application	:	Helps to relieve tension, uncontrolled anger, stress, anxiety, rapid heart rate, rapid breathing. Useful ion high blood pressure, menopause, PMT, insomnia, impotence, frigidity, scalp conditioner. Useful for skin care.
Precaution	:	Avoid using after consuming alcohol or before driving. Use in moderation. It may cause headache and nausea when taken in excess.

■

7

Simple Body Massage Step-By-Step

Just before you begin your massage check that your hands are clean and your nails fairly short with no jagged edges. Take off any rings if you wear them. You will find if you use aromatherapy oils regularly that your nails strengthen and your hands become smoother and more supple. Also, check with your massage partner to make sure there are no reasons to stop you going ahead.

The Feet

Probably the most neglected part of our bodies, feet deserve a loving massage from time to time. Make sure your partner is warm and comfortable. Uncover one foot by folding back the towel or blanker. Now pour a little of your chosen oil into the palm of one hand. Rub your hands together to evenly distribute the oil. Now you are ready to begin.

1. Enclose the foot between both hands (one on top, one underneath), then gently slide your hands off the foot coming forward to the toes. This movement should be slow and soothing. Repeat four or five times.
2. Gently circle around the ankles using your thumbs. This area can be tender, so go easy.
3. Rub over the top of the foot with your thumbs in little circles, coming down from the andkle area to the toes. Repeat three or four times.
4. Now rub each toe with the same little circular movements.
5. Rotate each toe twice in each direction.
6. Gently pull each toe between finger and thumb.

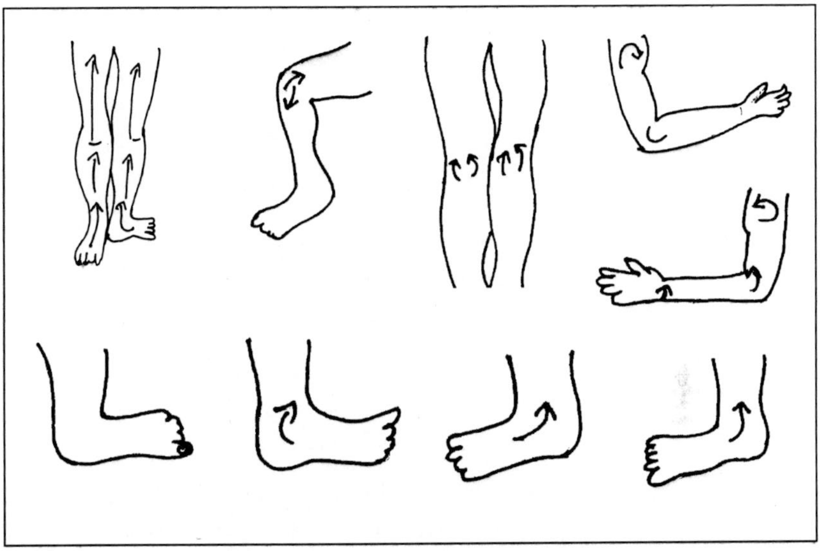

7. Zigzag down the sole of the foot from toes to heel with your thumbs overlapped.
8. Enclose the foot in your hands then rub them in opposite directions, to create frictions. This is very warming.
9. Hold the foot firmly and slowly rotate the ankle clockwise then anti-clockwise. Repeat a couple of times.
10. Repeat step 1.

Once complete, wrap the foot up again for warmth and repeat the movements on the other foot. By now your massage partner will be feeling more relaxed and at ease with your touch.

The Lower Legs and Knees

Warm a little oil in your hands.

1. With one hand behind the other, smooth the oil on to the front of the leg, starting at the top of the foot and working up to the knee. This movement distributes the oil and soothes and relaxes the whole area.

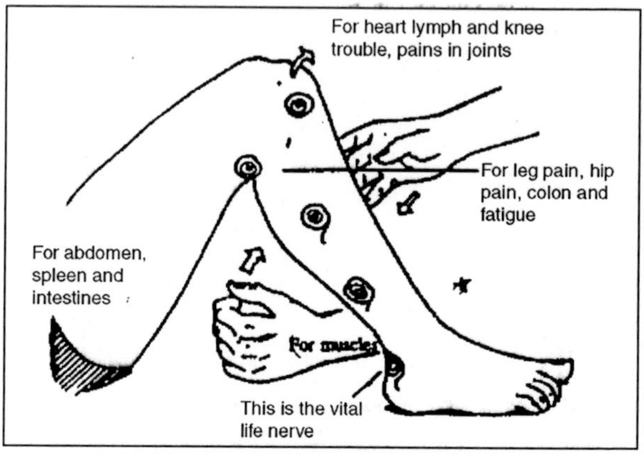

Lower Leg Massage

2. Rub acroos the front of the leg using both hands to create frictions. This increases the blood circulation to the area and reduces aches and pains.
3. Lift the leg up so the knee is bent. Squeeze and relax rhythmically down the muscles of the calf from knee to ankle. Repeat several times. Put the leg down.
4. Work around the kneecap in little circular motions with both hands. Be careful not to use too much pressure.
5. Now using your thumbs gently slide them around each side of the kneecap.
6. Stretch out your thumbs from your fingers to create an arch. Sweep over the whole knee using alternate hands several times.

Now Wrap up the lower leg and proceed to the thigh.

The Upper Legs

1. Apply oil as for trhe lower leg.
2. Glide up the leg from knee to groin, using one hand behind the other. This movement should be fairly slow and rhythmical. Make sure your movements cover the whole of the thigh area. Repeat four to five times.
3. Stroke the upper inner thigh diagonally from knee to groin hand over hand. Repeat four or five times.

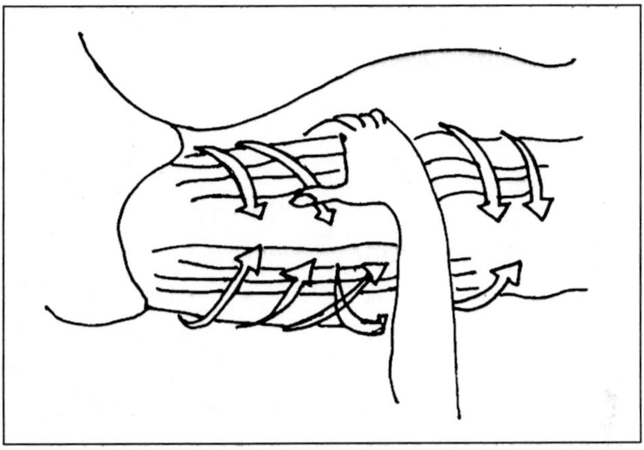

Upper Leg Massage

4. Squeeze and release rhythmically first along the inner thigh from knee to groin, then along the outer thigh.
5. Using your knuckles rake quickly up from the knee to the groin, taking in the whole thigh area. This is a friction movement and increases the surface blood circulation. You'll notice the skin colours quite quickly and feels warmer to the touch.
6. Uncover the lower leg, then effleurage the whole leg from foot to groin as in step 2.
7. Finish off by enclosing the foot in your hands a couple of times. Cover the leg then repeat all the movements on the other one.

By now you'll find your hands have become more sensitive to your partner and you'll notice differences in the skin texture and muscle tone.

The Hands and Arms

1. Smooth on the oil as before. When working on the arm it's easier to effleurage with one hand only, using the other to hold the arm steady.
2. Bend the arm at the elbow. Massage around the wrist with little thumb circles using both hands.

3. Work down from the wrist to the ends of the fingers using little thumb circles. Repeat five times.
4. Stretch each finger, then thumb, in turn between your finger and thumb.
5. Rotate the fingers and thumb first clockwise then anti-clockwise.
6. Turn the hand over and rub gently along the solar plexus (from centre wrist down the palm to the middle finger) using alternate thumbs. This is calming to the nervous system.

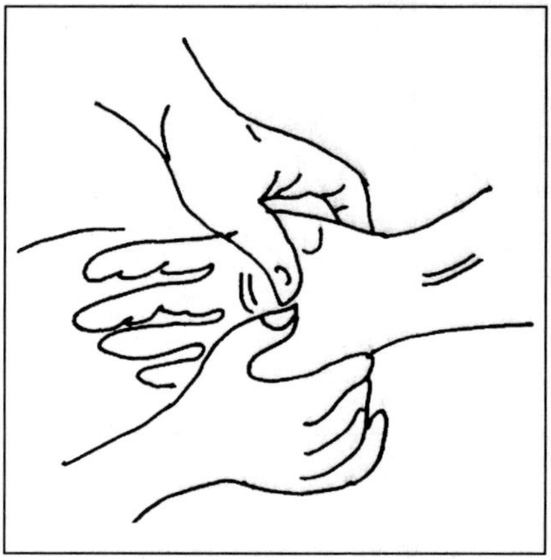

Palm Massage

7. Rotate the hand at the wrist clockwise then anti-clockwise. To do this lock your fingers into your partner's.
8. Turn the hand over and work on the inside of the wrist up to the elbow using alternate sweeping movements. Repeat four or five times.
9. Bend the arm at the elbow and bring the lower arm up and across the chest. Squeeze all along the upper arm from elbow to shoulder using both hands.

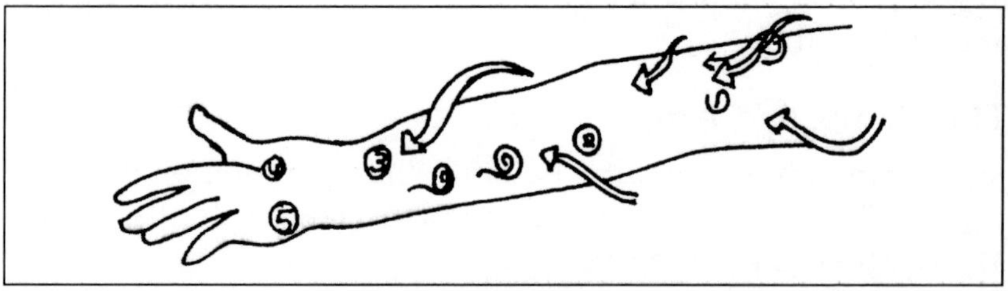

Arm Massage

10. Bring the arm back down to the side then effleurage the whole area from hand to shoulder four or five times. Cover the arm and repeat on the other side.

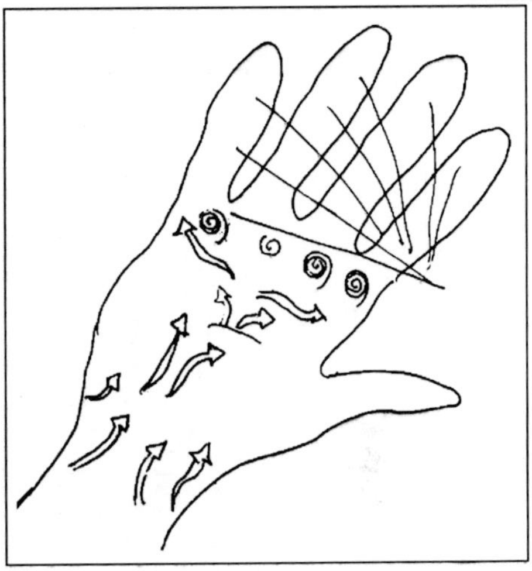

Palm Massage

The Abdomen

The abdomen is a soft area protecting vital organs, so please be gentle. Fold the towel or blanket down to expose the area from just below the breasts to a couple of inches (centimetres) below the navel.

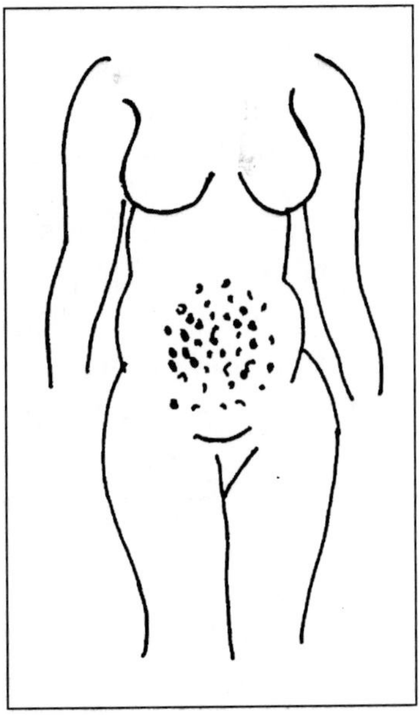

Abdominal Massage

1. Apply oil, starting just under the rib-cage, working down and out towards the waist. Be careful to keep your hands relaxed and contoured to your partner. Poking fingers feel very uncomfortable here.
2. With one hand on top of the other iron around the lower abdomen in large circles. Keep the pressure light and even.
3. Fan your hands out and work from the navel out to

the waist. Slide your hands under the waist then gently pull them back round to the front again. Repeat several times.

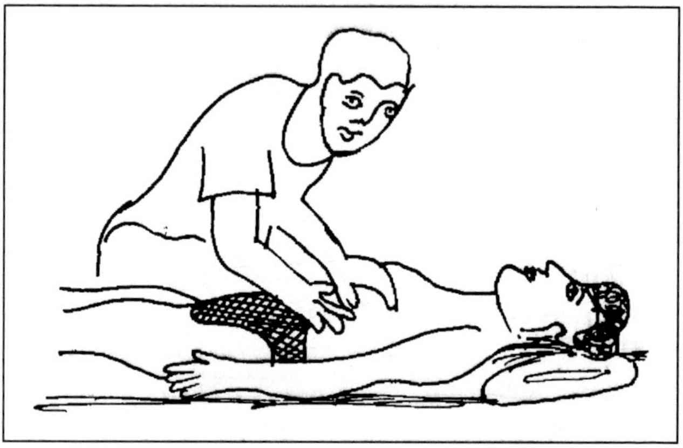

4. Stroke diagonally with alternate hands from the waist down to below the navel, first on the left side, then on the right.
5. Stroke down from the solar plexus to the navel, one hand behind the other, to finish off this area.

The Backs of the Legs

1. Effleurage oil as for the front of the legs but working from the foot right up to the top of the thigh. Repeat four of five times.
2. Bend the leg at the knee, supporting it with one hand. Stroke firmly down the calf, across behind the knee, then back up to the foot several times keeping your hands contoured to the leg. Put the leg down.
3. Work up the calf to the knee, using little circles. Repeat several times to cover the whole calf.
4. Using your index and middle fingers, make small circular movements behind the knee. Be careful not to press too hard.

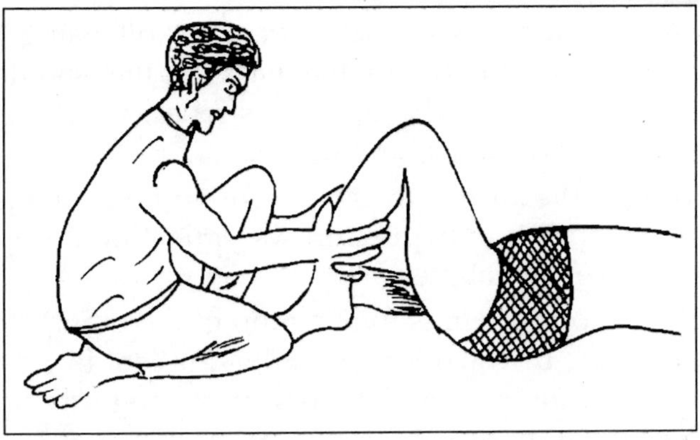

5. Squeeze rhythmically along the inner thigh from the knee upwards. Repeat on the outer thigh, doing each movement several times.

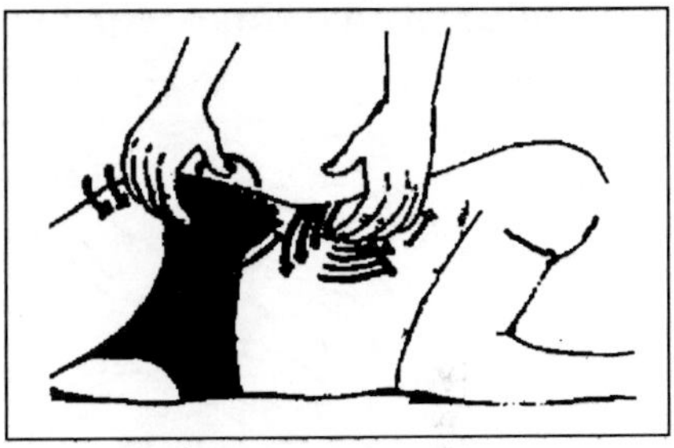

Hip and Side Massage

6. Diagonally stroke from the inner knee upwards and across the thigh. Repeat several times.
7. Finish by effeuraging the whole leg several times, from foot to thigh. Wrap up and repeat on the other leg.

The Back

Don't be at all surprised if your massage partner dozes off at this point. Back massage is extremely soothing and relaxing and great for relieving stress and tension.

Uncover the back to just show the buttock crease. At this point it is a good idea to place a small rolled-up towel under your partner's forehead otherwise he or she will have to turn his or her head sideways or end up with a squashed nose through which it is difficult to breathe.

1. Starting at the lower back effleurage oil using both hands. Work slowly up the back to the shoulders, pressing gently on the upward strokes, releasing the pressure as you come back down.
2. Starting at the base of the spine work up on either side, using gentle thumb pressure or little thumb circles. Repeat five or six times.
3. With reinforced hands (one on top of the other) sweep up the spine then work around the shoulder blades in a figure-of-eight movement. Repeat the figure-of-eight four or five times.
4. Now work around each shoulder blade individually, still with reinforced hands, in a circular motion. Repeat four of five times each side. You may feel knots (little

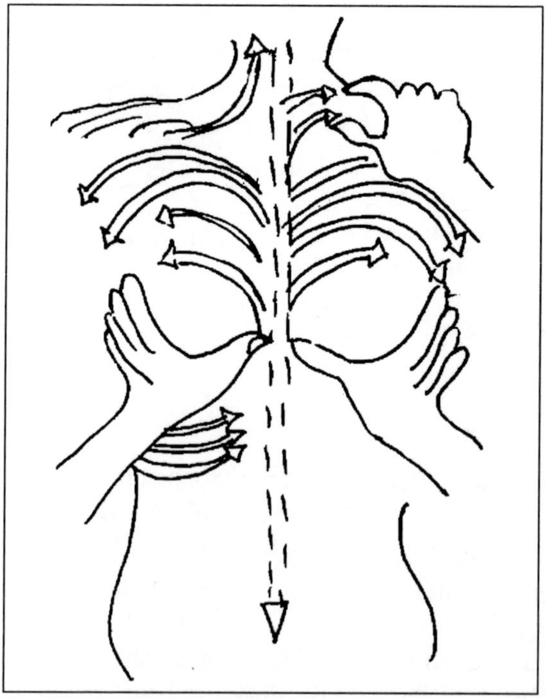

Upper Back Massage

bumps) around the shoulder blades. These are an indication of tension, and massage here gives great relief.

5. Work around the shoulder blades with your thumbs, helping to break down the knots and bumps. Allow your partner to be your guide as these areas can be tender.
6. Squeeze along the top of the shoulders from the neck out, using your fingers and thumbs. Repeat four to five times on each side.
7. Stroke up the back of the neck and out to the ears, using your thumbs.
8. Stand at your partner's head and sweep your hands down the centre back, across the top of the buttocks, then firmly pull up at the sides. Repeat five times.

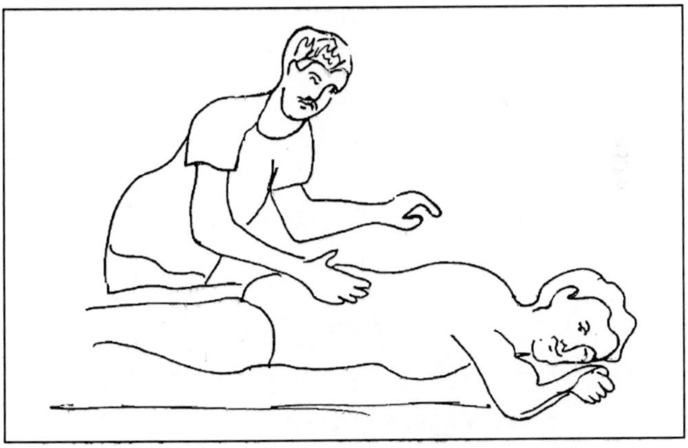

9. Move to your partner's side and rub backwards and forwards over the whole back with frictions to warm the area.
10. Make thumb circles out from just above the buttock crease round towards the hips. This area can often be tender and massage here is soothing. Repeat several times.

11. Effleurage the whole back.
12. Gently stroke up the spine, hand over hand, several times, allowing your touch to get lighter and lighter.

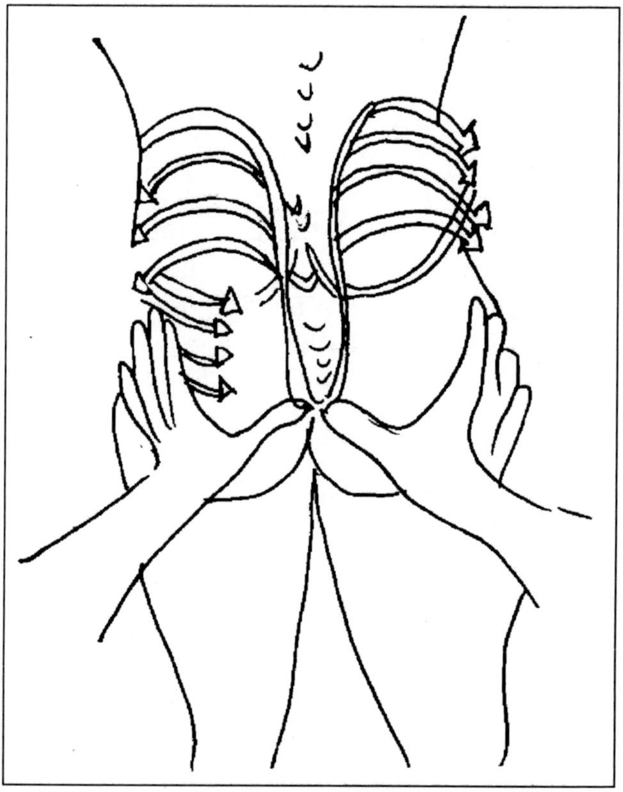

Lower Back Massage

13. Finish by gently holding your partner. Place one hand at the base of the spine, the other at the base of the neck. Hold this position and feel the warmth build up under your hands. After approximately one minute gently lift your hands off. Cover your partner over.

By now, he or she might be snoozing!

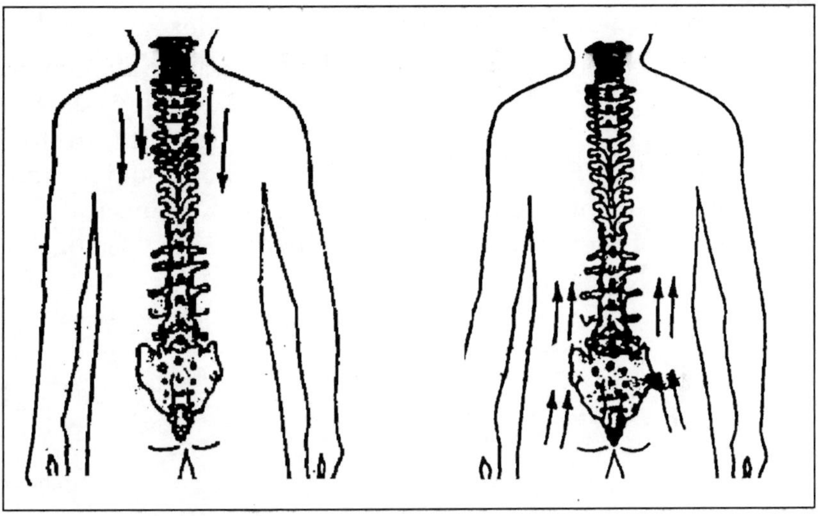

THE SHOULDERS AND NECK

If your partner is feeling very tense, and you haven't time to give a full body massage, working on the shoulders and neck will still offer great relief. For this your partner should be lying on his or her back. Uncover the chest by folding down the towel or blanket.

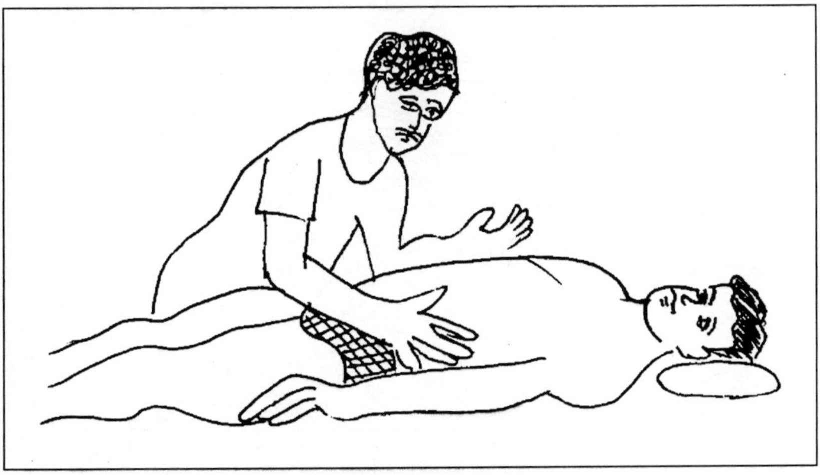

1. Apply oil to your partner's chest, shoulders and neck.
2. Begin effleuraging by placing both hands on the upper chest, fingers facing towards each other. Now, slowly pull your hands across the chest and out to the shoulders. Curve your hands round the shoulders and under them, then bring your hands in to meet at the back of the neck. Stroke up the neck to the base of the skull, Repeat four or five times.

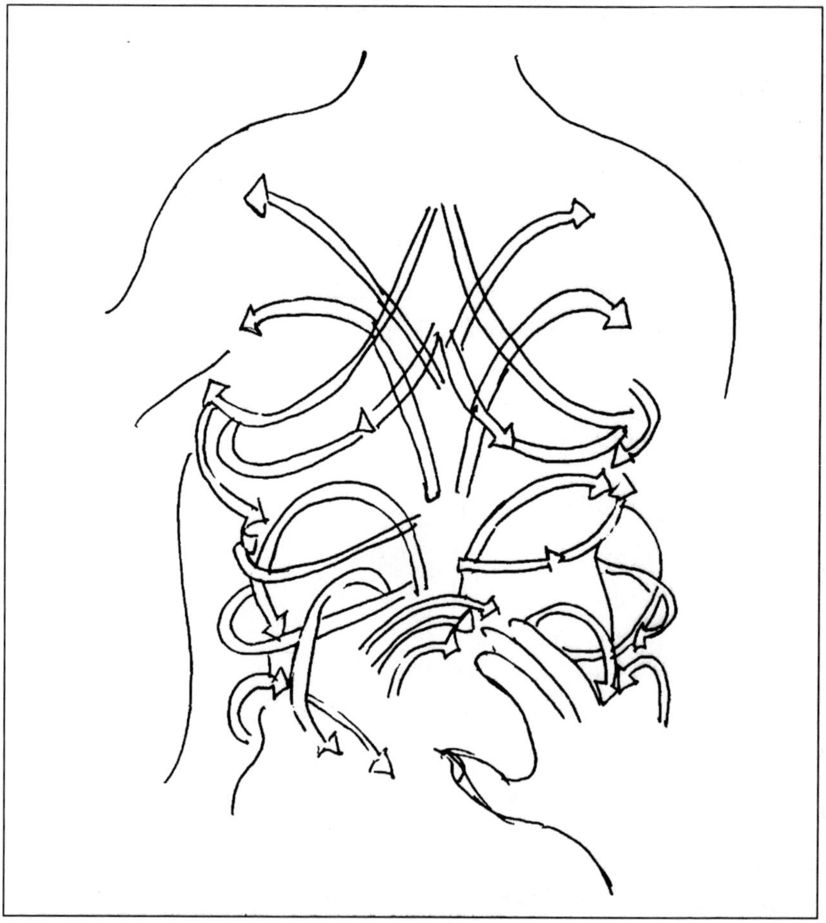

Front Body Massage

3. Gently knuckle the chest and shoulders in the sequence shown in the diagram. To knuckle make your hands into relaxed fists, and move the knuckles in circular movements. This sounds more difficult than it is.
4. Gently turn your partner's head to one side. Stroke along the top of the shoulder and the side of the neck with your first three fingers. Repeat three times.
5. Repeat the above sequence, but circle your fingers this time. Do this three times.
6. Turn your partner's head to the other side and repeat movements 4 and 5. Return the head to the centre.
7. Slide your hands down your partner's back as far as you can comfortably reach. Find the groove each side of the spine with your fingers. Pull your hands up the spine with a little pressure on the groove each side. Repeat three times.

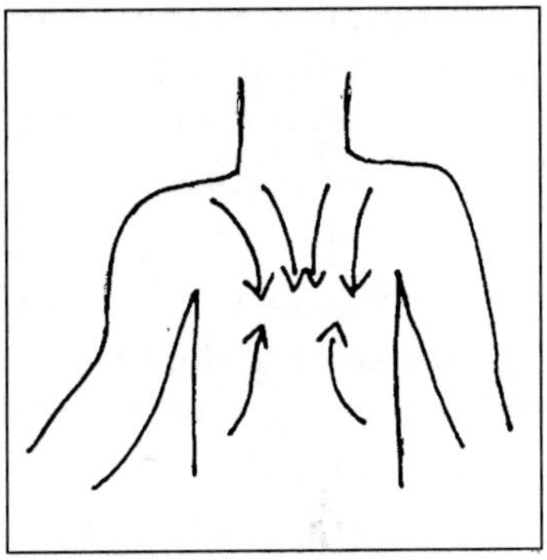

8. Now you are going to stretch the neck—these movements stretch out the muscles of the shoulders and neck and ease tension. If your partner is relaxed you'll find you will take all the weight of the head. If he or she is tense, go easy and make the movements slow and gentle. You don't want any pulled muscles.
9. Cup both hands unde your partner's head, your fingers resting in the base of the skull. Lift the head slightly, then gently pull towards you. Lower the head slowly, then repeat.
10. Hold the back of the head in one hand and move it slowly towards the left shoulder while gently pressing down on the right shoulder with your other hand. Bring the head back to the centre and then repeat on the other side.
11. Finish with some effleurage movements as you begin.

The Face and Scalp

Until you've had the pleasurable experience of a face massage you probably won't have realised how much tension we hold in our faces. Think of frowning—this is caused by muscle action, and these muscles tire just as much as those of any other part of the body. A caring face massage can smooth away some of this tension, leaving us looking (and feeling) more at ease and relaxed.

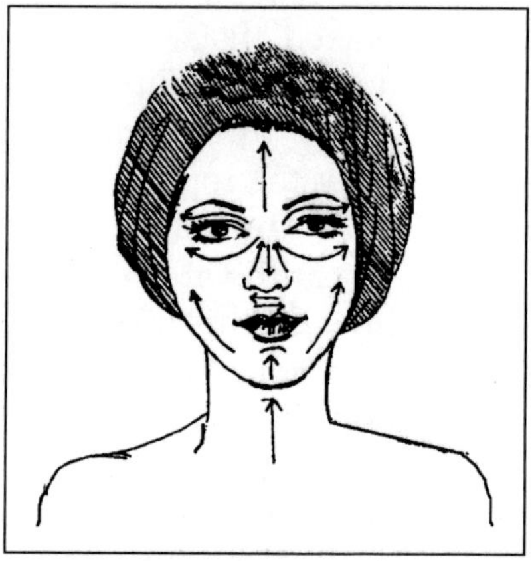

Face Care

Offer to take your partner's hair off the face with a headband, as it will inevitably get a little only around the hairline during the massage. Be careful not to use too much oil on the face or you'll find it difficult to massage specific areas without slipping.

Encourage your partner to close his or her eyes, so as to focus on your touch. Also, it can be disconcerting to have someone staring up at you, especially as a novice.

1. Begin by stroking up each side of the jawline to the forehead. Repeat four or five times.
2. Slowly stroke the forehead rhythmically with the flat of your hand from just above the brows to the hairline.
3. Starting at the centre hairline slide your thumbs out to the side, applying gentle pressure. Move down the forehead slightly and repeat. Continue this outward stroking pressure until you reach the eyebrows.
4. Now place the heel of each hand on the centre forehead and slide out to the sides. Repeat three times.
5. Place the first two fingers of each hand on the temples and circle gently for a minute or two, applying a little pressure.

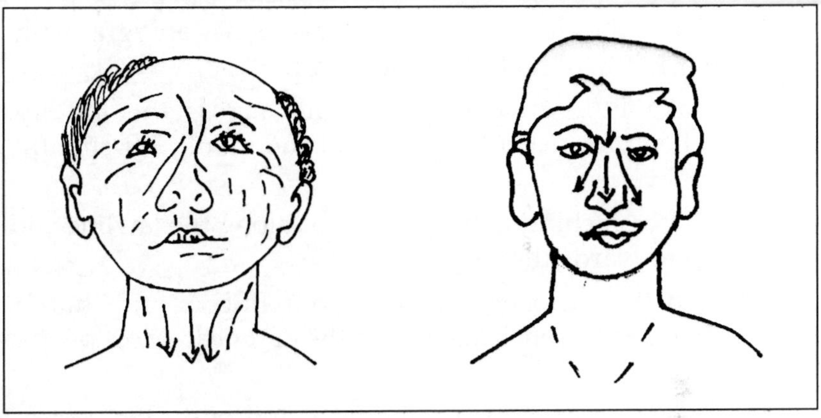

All the above movements help to relieve a headache. Try lavender oil for your massage, as I've found it can ward off a headache if used in time.

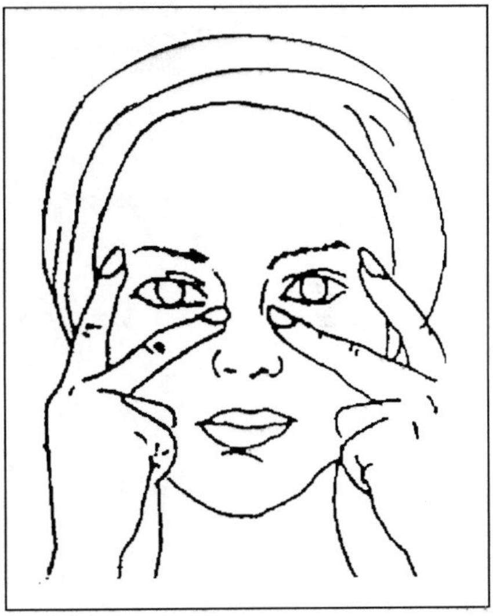

Eye Massage

6. Place your thumbs on your partner's inner eyebrows and slide out to the sides. Repeat three times.
7. With your index finger and thumb gently pull along the brow bone. Repeat three times.
8. Stroke gently over the eyelids with your ring fingers, from the inner to the outer corners. Repeat three times.
9. Alternately stroke down the nose with your thumbs, then gently rub round the nose tip and nostrils. Be careful not to press hard on the nostrils.

10. Stroke the cheeks across the cheekbones and gradually work down the face to the chin.
11. Make little circular movements across the top lip. When you reach the corner of the mouth lift slightly, then repeat.
12. Make pinching move-ments out along the jawline and up to-wards the ears.
13. Rub the earlobes bet-ween your fingers and thumb, then gently pinch all around the outer ear. Most people love this.
14. Sweep your hands up the neck and on to the cheeks. Hold, then repeat.
15. Finish by stroking the forehead, getting lighter and lighter until you bring your hands off.

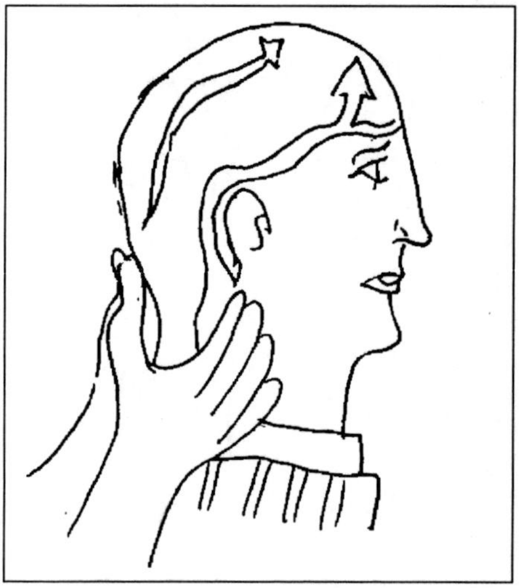

Scalp Movements

1. Remove your partner's headband. Bring your hands up the side of the face to the forehead, then rake them through the hair. Re-peat several times.

2. 'Glue' your fingers onto the scalp and move it around against the skull. Move your fingers to a different position and repeat this process until all the scalp has been covered.
3. Rub vigorously over the scalp, as if shampooing the hair.
4. Take little bunches of hair all over the scalp and tug gently. This feels lovely and really stimulates the scalp.
5. Repeat step 1 to finish off.

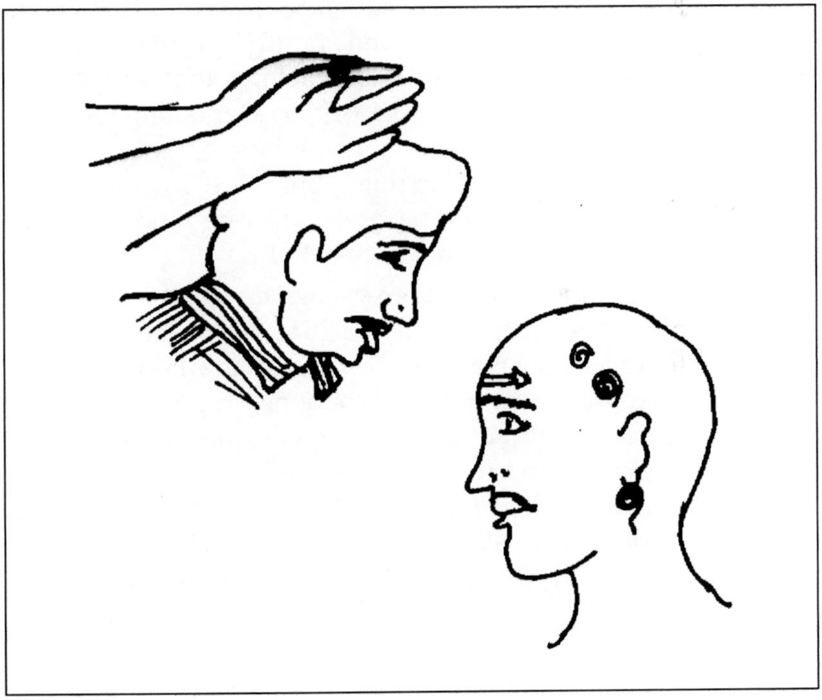

■

8

Wonderful Treatment Therapy—Shirodhara

Shirodhara means to pure medicated oil on head in a stream.

Now-a-days the problems of headache, high blood pressure, heart diseases, grey hair, etc. are very common. Financial, professional, social and family problems affect human life much. A tired body and aching limbs crave for attention at the end of day's hard work or after a long journey. At this time a hot or cold bath depending on the weather conditions brings great relief to them. But there is also another way to relieve such aches and pains. It is through massage and pressure. Shirodhara technique is a part of it.

In Ayurved, much importance was given to oil massage to protect health. The parts of a machine are oiled to work properly. In the same way the organs of the body require massage with oil to assist in their functions properly. Massage on head is much important as the mind controls all the organs of the body and then functions. Oil massage helps in the functions of the mind. It has been developed in Shirodhara. Mind and soul, which make a man active, reside in human brain according to Ayurved. Brain is their work-spot. It is the brain which controls all the functions of the body. Shirodhara is the best technique to keep the mind healthy.

Method

The body of the patient is massaged with oil at first. Then the patient is laid on a special table made for Shirodhara. Shirodhara is poured on his forehead and head. His eyes covered with cotton pads.

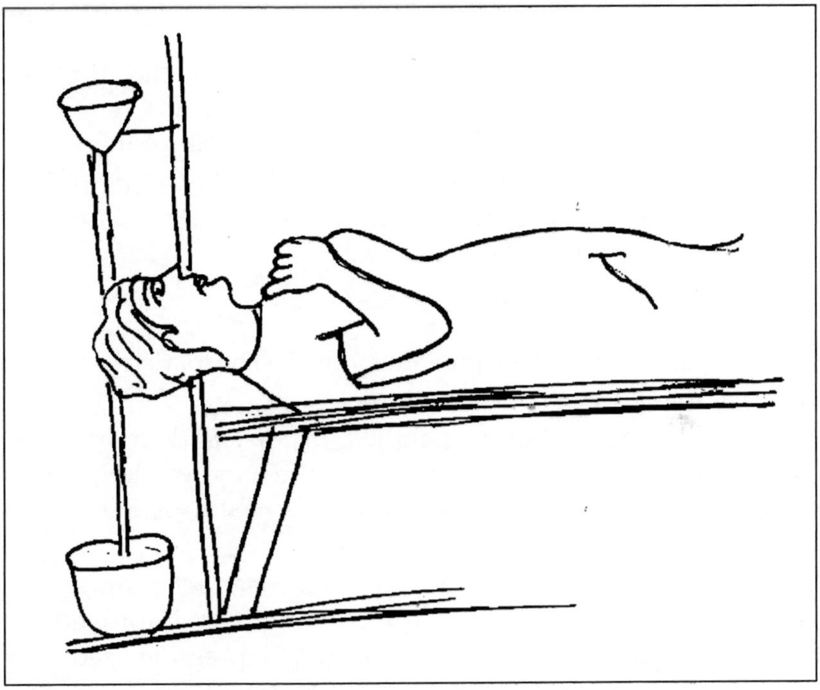

A special pot is made to keep oil. This pot is broad on the above side and small on the lower side. There is a small hole in the bottom of the pot. If this pot is made of gold, iron or earth its effect is better. Now-a-days iron or copper pots are used more. This pot is tied with a strong string 4 to 5 inches above the head of the patient lying on the table.

Now the pot is filled with medicated oil and its stream starts falling over the head of the patient. The stream of oil should fall over the mid of forehead of the patient. An attendant standing nearby takes special care of it. The falling oil over the forehead passes through a pipe and it is collected in a pot kept under the table for this purpose. This oil is again poured in the pot tied above the head of the patient. The process Shirodhara should not be discontinued before time.

Oil for Shirodhara

Medicines and oil are selected according to the diseases and nature of the patient. Ayurvedic medicines and herbs are boiled in mustard or til oil. This oil is used for Shirodhara.

Oil prepared with Dashmool medicines is used in Vat problems and oil prepard with Majeeth and Anantmool medicines is used in Pitta problems.

Time for Dhara

It should be done in morning hours. The patient should take rest for sometime after the process.

Benefits: Shirodhara pacifies brain and mind. It strengthens the senses. The senses and the mind work through the brain. The best way to improve the health of the mind, brain and senses is Shirodhara.

Its effects are good in relieving headache and Vat problems. Hearing power, voice and eyesight are improved by it. Tension, discomfort, despair, anger, depression, sadness and other mental agonies disturb the balance of the Vat which results in headache, greying of hair, falling of hair, insomnia, etc. Shirodhara is the best treatment has been adopted by a majority of patients in Kerala. Foreigners visit Kerala every year in large number to get relief in their diseases by Shirodhara and other techniques of massage.

■

9

Deep Cleansing by Facial Massage/Masks and Face Packs

Atleast once a week, a deep cleansing routine is a must for a clear complexion. Cleanse your face using a cleanser. Apply massage oil or cold cream and follow this with a facial massage.

Facial Massage

Facial massage revives and conditions your skin. It helps to raise your skin's temperature, thereby, improving the blood circulation. A facial massage also soothes and eases away tensions present in the facial muscles.

A massage is necessary for all skin types. As you grow older gracefully, massage takes a prominent role. Massage done with the right techniques, helps to tone and firm up sagging muscles.

Use a hair band to tie up your hair neatly, away from your face. Apply a good cream liberally all over face and neck.

Facial massage always begins at the base of your throat. Move towards the chin using fingers of one hand followed in quick succession with the fingers of the other hand.

Using the first and second finger, tap all over face and neck. Press thumbs under the middle of the chin line and gently stroke outward, towards the end of the jawline. Push your chin gently upwards using both hands. Move upwards on either side of your mouth and work your way towards your ear lobes. Massage your nose with small, upward movements on either side of the nose. Now move towards the centre of eyebrows and move around the eye using a circular movement. Move vertically from brows to hairline.

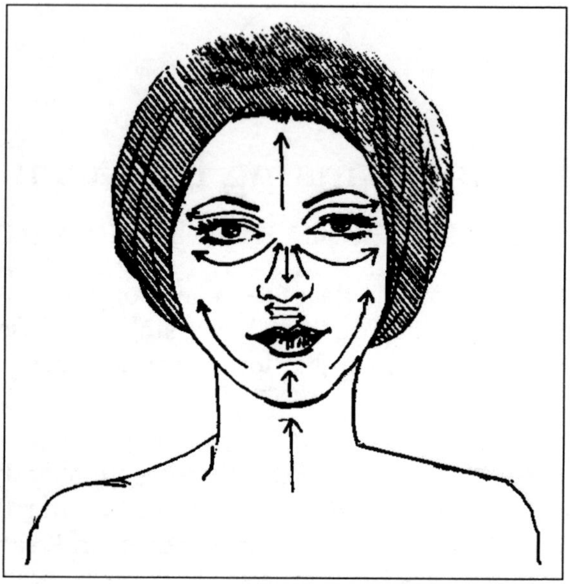

Face Care

Massage temples with slight pressure using small circular movements. Repeat this movement 4 times each. Allot extra time for problem areas like a lined forehead.

Steam Facial

Steaming dilates the pores. Steam penetrates and deep cleanses the pores, bringing to the surface all the hidden grease and dirt. Steaming brings out a lovely glow on your face instantly, an effective treatment for a fresh shine on face.

Skin the weekly steaming process, if you have a dry, sensitive skin.

- ☞ Use the steam electric unit for steaming. Alternatively, you may use a basin filled with steaming hot water.
- ☞ You may like to add herbs or flowers to the hot water. Steep herbs/flowers in hot water for five minutes. However, if you have a lot of blackheads, throw in a few crystals of camphor instead of herbs.

☞ Bend over basin.

☞ Cover your head with a towel to trap the steam inside.

☞ Close your eyes and hold your head as close to the steam as you can without any discomfort.

☞ Breathe in the vapours. The aroma of the herbs will stimulate a soothing, relaxed feeling.

☞ Allow the vapours to streak down your face.

☞ Once your pores are dilated with the steaming process, wipe the face with a tissue or a damp cotton wool.

☞ Remove blackheads by gently pressing it, using a blackhead remover and sterilised cotton wool.

☞ Splash with warm water and follow it with icy cold water.

☞ You may apply a face mask now.

FACE MASK

Masks are excellent beauty revivers and they provide the skin with an instant wonder filip. Masks lend a smooth complexion to the user. Masks are more effective after a steam facial.

Mask guidelines

Carefully select the masks best suited to your skin type and remember.

☞ If you are treating your skin for the first time with a face mask, you may find a few blemishes a week later. This indicates that the treatment is working well.

☞ Masks must always be used on a clean skin.

☞ Apply a face mask when skin is warm.

☞ Mask application must be avoided around the eyes and mouth.

☞ For dry, sensitive and combination skin types, the mask may be washed off after ten minutes.

- ☞ Oily skin needs a mask for a full fifteen minutes before rinsing off.
- ☞ Vary treatments from season to season.
- ☞ Once you know your skin type and its limitations, you can decide on a face mask made from a wide variety of flowers, fruits, vegetables and dairy products.
- ☞ Fortify your skin with some of natures most amazing beauty ingredients

Avocado Mask

Avocado Mask is a perfect mask for dry skin.

Ingredients : ½ teaspoon honey or safflower oil and
1 egg yolk.
¼ teaspoon honey or safflower oil.

Method : Mask avocado well. Add beaten egg yolk and honey.

Application : Apply on skin and rinse off after 15 minutes.

Carrot Mask

Carrot contains plenty of vitamin A and is excellent for sensitive skin.

Ingredients : ½ carrot
¼ teaspoon honey

Method : Grate carrot. Extract the juice and stir in honey.

Application : Pat on skin. Leave on for 10-15 minutes. Rinse off.

Potato Mask (is an ideal mask for dry skin)

Ingredients : ½ tablespoon curds
1 teaspoon curd

Method : Add curd to well grated potato and mix well.

Application : Apply on face and let it dry for 15 minutes before washing off.

Oatmeal mask have softening as well whitening properties. Use oatmeal grains as exfoliating masks.

Simple Oatmeal Mask

Ingredients	:	1½ tablespoon oatmeal A little milk water
Method	:	Oatmeal is soaked in milk and water for 15 minutes
Application	:	Apply as a mask.

Tomato Mask for Oily Skin

Ingredients	:	1 Tomato Rind of ½ lemon A dash of lemon juice
Method	:	Mask tomato and mix with very finely grated rind and add a dash of lemon juice.
Application	:	Put on face and rinse off after 10 minutes with warm water.

Kaolin and Wheatgerm Mask

Ingredients	:	1 tablespoon oatmeal ½ teaspoon wheat germ powder 1 teaspoon kaolin
Method	:	Soak oatmeal in lukewarm water for 10 minutes. Add wheatgerm and kaolin.
Application	:	Apply all over the face and neck and leave on for 15 minutes. Wash off with tepid water.

Wheatgerm Mask

Ingredients	:	½ tablespoon wheatgerm ½ tablespoon oatmeal 1 teaspoon olive oil 1 teaspoon fresj cream.

Method : Combine wheatgerm and oatmeal. Add to it olive oil and fresh cream to make a thick paste.

Application : Apply evenly and rinse off after 10 minutes.

Cooling Mask

Ingredients : ½ tablespoon oatmeal
½ tablespoon wheat germ
1 teaspoon milk powder
1 teaspoon sandal wood powder
1 teaspoon barley powder
½ teaspoon fenugreek powder
1 teaspoon kaolin

Method : Soak oatmeal in water for 10 minutes and combine all ingredients. Use just enough water to make into paste and apply. Leave it on for 15 minutes before washing it off.

Revitalising Mask

Ingredients : 1 tablespoon brewer's yeast
2 capsule of vitamin E
1 capsule of vitamin D
1 capsule of vitamin A

Method : Prick a pin into each capsule, squeeze contents and add in yeast and mix well.

Application : Apply mask and leave on 30 minutes. Rinse off.

Yeast Mask (for oily skin)

Ingredients : 1 tablespoon brewer's yeast
2 tablespoon yoghurt

Method : Make a light, thin mixture combining the above ingredients.

Application	:	Apply all over the skin and allow it to dry for 20 minutes. Rinse off with lukewarm water, splash cold water and pat dry.

Egg Mask

Ingredients	:	1 egg lemon juice or honey
Method	:	Beat one egg and add 1 teaspoon honey for dry skin or 1 teaspoon of lemon juice of you have an oily skin.
Application	:	Apply all over face for 15 minutes. Wash off thoroughly.

Cucumber Mask (for sluggish and tired face)

Ingredients	:	½ cup mashed cucumber 1 white of an egg 2 teaspoon skimmed milk powder
Method	:	Mix well to make a smooth paste.
Application	:	Apply all over the face and leave on for 20 minutes before rinsing with warm water. Use chilled water for the final rinse. Blot dry.

Special Aloe vera Mask

Ingredients	:	1 small aloe leaf 1 tablespoon honey 1 teaspoon kaolin
Method	:	Cut open the aloe leaf scrape out the fleshy portion. Liquidise aloe pulp for 1 minutes. Add honey and kaolin and whisk for ½ minutes. This is ideal for softening and toning. This mask is suitable for all types of skin. Replace honey with lime juice for oily skin.

Winter Mask (ideal for winter dryness)

Ingredients : 1 tablespoon brewer's yeast
2 tablespoon or more distilled water

Method : Make a smooth paste of the yeast and water.

Application : Apply thickly all over face and leave on for 15 minutes. Wash off with tepid water.

Honey Mask

Ingredients : 1 tablespoon Fuller's earth
1 tablespoon honey
1 teaspoon rose water
10 drops of orange juice

Method : Mix all the ingredients together

Application : Apply on face and wash off after 15 minutes.

Oatmeal Mask for Oily Skin

Ingredients : 1 tablespoon oatmeal powder
½ tablespoon lemon juice
3 teaspoon of milk

Method : Mix all ingredients together to a smooth consistency.

Application : Apply on oily facial skin evenly and wash off after 15-20 minutes.

Parsley Mask (for combination skin)

Ingredients : 1 bunch parsley leaves
1 tablespoon honey

Method : Chop parsley leaves finely and put in liquidiser with a little water for 3-5 seconds. Remove and strain out the juice. Mix with honey.

Application : Use all over the face. After 20 minutes rinse well with cold water. Pat dry.

Honey and Egg Mask (to give skin tone and elasticity)

Ingredients : 1 egg
1 tablespoon sesame oil
1 teaspoon honey

Method : Put only yolk in the blender on low speed. Slowly add sesame seed oil. Add honey and egg white and continue blending on low speed until the mixture reaches the texture for application.

Application : Apply on face and wash off thoroughly with water after 20 minutes. You will see the difference almost immediately.

Honey Face Mask

Ingredients : ½ tablespoon honey
½ tablespoon barley
1 egg white

Method : Mix barley with honey and add in frothy egg white to form a smooth paste.

Application : Apply liberally and evenly on entire face, leaving out eyes and mouth area. Allow it to dry for 10 minutes. Wash with warm water. Finish off with a splash of icy cold water.

Starch Mask (to make enlarged pores less evident and restore healthy glow to cheeks)

Ingredients : 1 tablespoon potato starch or wheat starch or corn starch
Warm water

Application : Massage your face gently with little olive oil. Then apply starch mask on the face and neck. Leave the mask on for 20 minutes and rinse off thoroughly with warm water.

Barley Face Mask

Ingredients : 1 tablespoon barley powder
1 tablespoon of milk
1 teaspoon of lemon juice

Method : Mix the first two ingredients together. Add enough lemon juice to make a thick paste.

Application : Apply on face and rinse off after 10 minutes.

Egg-cream Facial Mask (to revive skin tone)

Ingredients : 1 egg white
1 tablespoon cream
¼ teaspoon of castor sugar.

Method : Beat the egg white until it becomes white and fluffy, add cream and sugar. Best together.

Application : With a brush, apply a thick layer all over the face.
Leave on for 20 minutes and rinse off with warm water.

Masks for Problem Skin

Ingredients : 1 banana
2-3 tablespoon of milk

Method : Mash banana and add milk to make a paste.

Application : Apply all over the face and leave if for 15 minutes before washing it off with lukewarm water.

Olive Oil Mask (for blemishes)

Ingredients : ½ tablespoon of olive oil
¼ tablespoon of lemon juice

Method : Mix the ingredients together well.

Application : Apply the application to remain for 15 minutes before washing off.

Mint Mask (for blemishes)

Ingredients : 1 sprig mint leaves

1 teaspoon rose water.

Method : Wash and grind the mint leaves to a smooth paste using rose water.

Application : To be applied preferably overnight or leave on for a couple of hours before washing off.

Almond Mask

Ingredients : 4 almonds

2 tablespoon of milk

1 teaspoon orange juice

1 vitamin A capsule

Method : Soak almonds in water. Grind with milk and add orange juice. Squeeze contents of vitamin A capsule and mix well.

Application : Apply on face andneck. Leave on for 20 minutes before washing off.

All Purpose Mask

Ingredients : ½ barley powder

½ olive oil (if skin is dry)

1 teaspoon curd

1 teaspoon lemon juice

1 teaspoon carrot juice

1 teaspoon gelatine (dissolved in water)

2 teaspoon brewer's yeast powder

Method : Blend all the ingredients well.

Application : Apply over face and neck and rinse off thoroughly with cold water.

Here the fruit and vegetable juices supply the needed vitamins and minerals, barley supplies protein, yeast stimulates the flow of blood and curd cleanses the skin.

Raw Papaya Mask

Ingredients	:	A small piece of raw papaya
Method	:	Grate papaya finely and extract juice.
Application	:	Saturate cottonwool into the juice and apply over blemished skin. Wash off after fifteen minutes.

Yoghurt based Masks

Yoghurt may be combined with other ingredients to form various combination of mask.

Yoghurt is an excellent cleansing, softening as well binding agent. Yoghurt is suitable for all skin types. Hence you can combine yoghurt or buttermilk with other ingredients.

Prepare a mask suited for your skin.

- ☞ Yoghurt combined with tamato pulp serves as a good astringent.
- ☞ Yoghurt and mashed cucumber has a toing and freshing effect.
- ☞ Yoghurt and honey helps dry skin.
- ☞ Yoghurt can be combined with equal parts of Fuller's earth and dilluted with mint juice.
- ☞ When combined with crushed parsley leaves it makes an excellent mask for combination skin.
- ☞ Egg white with yoghurt softens the skin.

All yoghurt based mask, must be first washed off with warm water and finished off with a splash of cold water.

Moisturising or Softening Masks

These mask contain ingredients such as fruit juices and glycerine which improves the sin's ability to retain moisture and prevent loss of moisture from the skin.

Fruit based Mask

- ☞ Papaya mask is excellent to lend a healthy glow to the skin.
- ☞ Mash a small piece of papaya and spread over your face and neck. After a lapse of 15 minutes rinse it off with cold water.
- ☞ De-seed grapes and rub the pulp all over the face and rinse it off with cold water after 20 minutes.
- ☞ Mashed strawberries and peaches may also be used in the same way.

Remedies for Greasy Skin

Ingredients : 1 teaspoon of cucumber juice
½ teaspoon lemon juice
3 drops of rose water

Combine together and apply on face. Leave for 15 minutes before washing off.

Ingredients : 1 sprig of lettuce leaves
1 tablespoon rose water
½ teaspoon lemon juice

Guind to a paste lettuce leaves using rose water. Add lemon juice before application.

Ingredients : 1 tablespoon gram flour
2 tablespoon cucumber juice.

Method : Combine both the ingredients and apply evenly over entire face, leaving out eyes and mouth area. Wash off after 15 minutes using tepid water.

FACE PACKS

All skin types benefit from the deep-cleansing activities of a face pack. Face pack cleanses deep into the pores and actually freshens up the skin's texture.

Egg Face Pack

This face pack is especially beneficial to dry skin types.

Ingredients	:	1 egg yolk 1 teaspoon honey 1 tablespoon milk powder, rose water.
Method	:	Mix the ingredients together. Use rose water to achieve a paste form.
Application	:	Apply all over face and neck. Wash off water fifteen minutes using warm water.

Face Pack for Dry Skin

Ingredients	:	1 tablespoon of olive oil ½ lemon, 1 egg yolk.
Method	:	Extract the juice of the lemon, add olive oil and egg yolk. Mix well.
Application	:	Apply and leave on for fifteen minutes and wash off.

Fuller's Earth Face Pack (for oily, large-pored skin)

Ingredients	:	1½ tablespoon Fuller's earth 1½ tablespoon lemon juice ½ tablespoon honey
Method	:	Mix all ingredients together to form a paste.
Application	:	After application, wash after 15 minutes with lukewarm water

Winter Pack

Ingredients	:	1 tablespoon of wheat gram, olive oil
Method	:	Combine the above ingredients to make a paste.
Application	:	Apply over the face and relax for fifteen minutes. Wash off gently.

Facial Pack (ideal for dry skin)

Ingredients	:	1 teaspoon almond oil 1 teaspoon olive oil
Method	:	Mix both the oil together
Application	:	Apply over face and rinse off after fifteen minutes.

Banana Honey Pack

Ingredients	:	½ banana ½ tablespoon honey
Method	:	Mash banana well, add in honey and mix well.
Application	:	Apply well, all over face and rinse off after ten to fifteen minutes.

Honey Pack (for wrinkled skin)

Ingredients	:	1 egg white 2 tablespoon honey
Method	:	Mix all ingredients and make a thick paste.
Application	:	Apply the pack and relax on bed until dry. Wash off.

Moisturising—the landmark of good skin care

Moisturising forms a barrier between the skin and environmental conditions. Moisturiser helps to form a fine, protective layer that enables the skin to retain the Moisture it requires. Moisturising is essential for all types of skin including oily skin. Dry skin and ageing skin derive the maximum benefits from a moisturiser. Lack moisture on the skin causes skin to become dry and more prone to wrinkling.

Moisturisers come in two forms: liquid and cream. Rich, liquid and cream moisturisers take care of dry and wrinkled skin. A water-based, oil free moisturiser works best for oily skin.

Herbal moisturisers are very light. They not only hlp to protect the skin but also assist in evaporating excess of moisture.

Ideally, moisturisers are applied after thorough cleansing and toning of your skin. Moisturiser may be used before make-up to serve as a protective base. Use a moisturiser of light consistency, as it will assist your make-up to hold better. For dry skin, you may apply a moistriser even under a face pack. At night, dry skin requires a heavier moisturiser to feed your skin.

An excellent moisturiser protects skin from premature ageing due to sunlight and is a good occluder for depleting moisture balance. Apply extra moisturiser on your forehead, centre of brows and all over neck.

A few easy to make moisture creams with its gentle blend of waxes and oils. These specially formulated creams restore the skin's emollient feel.

Moisturising Cream

Ingredients : 4 tablespoons vegetable oil
2 teaspoon lenolin
2 teaspoon glycerine
1 teaspoon beeswax
1 teaspoon emulsifying wax
1¼ teaspoon borax
3 teaspoon water.

Method : Melt oil, wax and lanolin using the double boiling method. Heat water and borax until borax is completely dissolved. Stir in glycerine. Add very slowly, the borax, glycerine and water to the melted waxes while still under heat. Stir continuously with a wooden spatula until it is cool.

You may add a few drops of perfume when it is cold.

Moisturiser for Oily Skin

Ingredients : 1½ teaspoon almond oil
1 teaspoon lanolin
½ tablespoon olive oil
½ tablespoon emulsifying wax
2 teaspoon glycerine
6 tablespoons rose water.

Method : Melt waxes using double boiling method and add almond and olive oil. Stir in glycerine and hot rose water slowly. Continue to stir until the mixture is cold.

■

10

Nourishing Your Skin

For a supple, smooth complexion, nourishing is equally important. A good nourshing cream must be applied over face and neck to improve circulation before retiring.

For dry skin and ageing skin, you may take on a second application. After 40, the formulation of hormones and other vital elements slow down and this calls for a rich, nourishing cream to give your skin a more youthful appearance.

There are oil based as well as moisturing nourishing creams. Creams, lotions, skin foods, vitaminised creams and anti-wrinkle creams are all nourishing preparations.

Applying Cream

Using both your hands stroke gently working your way from throat to chin, to ears, brow to temples and eye area. Start from the outer corner of eye move towards the tear and move on to upper eyelids. Remove cream using the same technique.

Olive Oil Nourishing Cream

Ingredients : 3 tablespoons of olive oil
2 tablespoons of coconut oil
½ tablespoon beeswax
½ teaspoon borax
3 tablespoons water

Method : Heat the oil slightly. Heat and dissolve completely the borax in the water. Slowly add the heated Borax water to oil until the mixture becomes thick.

Vitaminised Nourishing Cream

Ingredients : 1 tablespoon beeswax
1 tablespoon emulsifying wax
3 vitamin E capsule
3 vitamin A capsule
½ teaspoon borax
½ teaspoon almond oil
1-2 drops of tincture of benzoin

Method : Melt waxes and lanolin by the double boiling method. Simultaneously, dissolve borax in warm water. Add the water to the wax. Beat until it cools slightly. Squeeze out oil from the capsules and add to mixture. Add a drop of benzoin and whisk until it thickens.

Orange Nourishing Cream

Ingredients : 1 tablespoon beeswax
2 tablespoon of olive oil
4 teaspoons of almond oil
1 teaspoons of emulsifying wax
2 teaspoons of lanolin
3 teaspoons of orange flower water
2-3 drops of tincture of benzoin

Method : Melt oils and waxes using the double boiling method. Add hot orange flower water and tincture of benzoin. Keep stirring till done.

Rich Lanolin Nourishing Cream

Ingredients : 2 teaspoon witch hazel
10 teaspoon of lanolin
2 tablespoon almond oil

Method : Melt lanolin by the double boiling method. Beat witchhazel almond oil and combine with lanolin. Store in an air-tight container.

Lanolin Nourishing Cream

Ingredients : 2 teaspoon of honey
6 teaspoon lanolin
2 tablespoon lecithin

Method : Mix together the ingredients and melt using the double boiling method. Add 7 tablespoons of warm water to it. Whisk continuously until it cools.

Effective Substitute for Cold Cream

Equal parts of lemon juice and glycerine is an excellent cold cream substitute that may be used at bed time.

Orange Nourishing Cream

Ingredients : 2 teaspoons of olive oil
2 teaspoon witch Hazel
2 tablespoon of fresh orange juice
2 tablespoon of glycerine
8 teaspoon of grated pears soap
4 tablespoons of cold water.

Method : Add water to the soap and heat over a low fire until the soap dissolves. Remove from heat. Add olive oil, glycerine, orange juice and witch hazel stirring continuously. Place back on low flame and stir until it begins to thickens. Transfer to a glass and allow it to settle for atleast 10 days before using it.

PORE SHRINKING TECHNIQUES

Oily skin requires more cleansing than creaming. Oily skinned persons won't, have to worry about sunning or wrinkles, neither will they be prone to a premature ageing look.

Oily skin has the disadvantage of perpetually shiny nose, a skin that hates make-up and of course, a tendency to large pores.

Large pored skin does not look lovely at close quarters. Large pores provide a base for blackheads and pimples.

Here are the oldest methods of shrinking large pores:

☞ Wash face with warm water and pure soap. Rinse off. Splash cold water and dry well with a coarse towel. Rub the fresh juice of lemon over entire face and allow it to dry. Wash off. Lemon juice acts as an astringent which clears and closes pores.

☞ Clean your face with warm water. Apply two tablespoons of milk of magnesi. Rinse off water twenty minutes with tepid water and finish off with a dash of cold water.

☞ Soak 5 almonds for an hour. Grind to a paste using 1 teaspoon of lemon juice. Leave for 15-20 minutes and rinse off with lukewarm water.

☞ On washed clean face, a pply white off egg and leave on for 25 minutes. Wash face using lukewarm water and follow with a cold water rinse.

☞ Saturate cotton wool with buttermilk, pat over face. Allow to dry before rinsing off.

☞ A combination of equal quantities of tomato juice and butter milk is also an excellent pore tightener.

☞ Extract the juice of lettuce leaves, add 2-3 drops of lemon juice and use over face. Wash off with cold water.

☞ Apricots combined with the pulp of tomato is an excellent pore shrinker.

☞ To the well beaten white of an egg. Add and mix well just a grain of camphor. Apply evenly for 20 minutes before rinsing off.

■

11

Acne and Pimples

There are a common inflammatory disorders of the sebaceous glands just below the skin surface and characterized by the recurring formation of black heads, white heads and pimples.

Acne

Primarily, acne occurs on the face but in some cases, it may be noticed by the back, shoulders, chest and arms.

Hormones—The culprits are at their peak of activity thus influencing the secretion of the sebaceous glands. The excess production of sebum causes breakouts that are highly incident during puberty and menstruation. At times, psychological stress causes acne.

Cleanse skin morning and night with milk home-made cleansers. Refrain from using facial scrub, when acne is severe. Stop picking your pimples and acne.

Diet—an important factor in acne.

Balanced nutrition and diet, skin hygiene, adequate sleep, exercise, fresh air and sunlight help in combating acne.

Carbohydrates and foods with a high fat content should be avoided from diet.

The high content of oxalic acid that is present in chocolates, coca and rhubarb inhibit the body's absorption of calcium. Since calcium maintains the acid-alkali balance of the body, it is important for a clear complexion.

Reducing salt intake in your diet also shows a remarkable improvement in complexion. Vitamins are necessary for your lovely, smooth skin.

Vitamin A is important for clear, healthy skin.

Vitamin B complex reduces facial greasiness and the formation of blackheads.

Combating Acne

- ☞ Saturate cotton wool in mint juice extract and apply every day.
- ☞ Apply crushed marigold leaves on acne.
- ☞ Boil and mash plums to get roughly eight teaspoons. Combine with 1 teaspoon of almond oil and apply.
- ☞ Make a smooth paste of Kasturi Turmeric and apply evenly on acne.
- ☞ Apply a mask made out of fresh neem leaves ground to a fine paste. Add a ¼ teaspoon of turmeric powder, sandal wood paste and gram flour. Let it dry completely before rinsing.

Banishing Pimples

- ☞ Swab face with camphor lotion on pimples daily. Wash off with medicated soap and lukewarm water.
- ☞ Grind mint leaves to extract pure juice. Apply generously and allow it to dry, before washing off.
- ☞ Sandal wood ground to a paste using undiluted cucumber juice may be used.
- ☞ One tablespoon of germ flour, half teaspoon of turmeric powder, one teaspoon of neem juice and enough milk to make a smooth consistency. Leave on for twenty minutes before washing off.
- ☞ Pimples can vanish overnight if you dot a little starch paste on the pimple at bedtime.

■

12

Whitening Complexion

The herbal way for those of us, who have not been blessed with a fair complexion, here are a few recipes to help to lighten your skin tone.

- A paste made out of sandalwood and rose water may be applied everyday.
- Turmeric paste combined with sandal wood paste makes your skin noticeably fairer.
- Cucumber juice is considered to be an excellent whitener.
- Coconut milk combined with equal quantities of cucumber juice may be applied as often as possible.
- Gently massage coconut water all over face and neck to lighten skin tone.
- Almonds ground to a paste using rose water or milk is said to make your skin fair.
- Make a paste using red sandalwood and rose water. This preparation not only whitens your complexion but also helps to fade away scars and blemishes on the skin's surface.

Complexion Sparklers

Put back a glowy shine on your face.

- Combine together equal quantities of salt and baby oil. Rub gently to slough away rough, dull skin.
- Boil neem leaves in water and allow to sleep before using it as a face wash.

- ☞ Use a cotton pad to apply undiluted orange juice all over face and neck.
- ☞ A beneficial substitute for hard water is soft water. Use it for a sparkling complexion.
- ☞ Splash face with icy cold water to which powdered nutmeg has been added.

Effective Methods for Removing Black and White Heads

- ☞ Rub face gently with pears soap and table salt. This helps to dislodge whiteheads. Rinse off with cold water.
- ☞ Use camphor BP crystals in the hot water used for steam facial.
- ☞ Cleanse your face with unboiled milk. Gently rub with a friction mitt dipped in milk to remove white as well as black heads.
- ☞ Apply a paste made out of Fuller's earth and rose water on face. When dry, rub with friction mitt to dislodge impurities.
- ☞ A solution made out of one and half cups of hot water and half a tablespoon of boric powder is an ideal concoction for blackheads. Saturate a face napkin in this hot solution and press on to face. Repeat. Extract blackheads with blackhead remove and sterilised cottonwool.
- ☞ Rub oatmeal paste (make wirh a little water) on face. Allow to dry for 15 minutes before washing off with cold water.
- ☞ After a facial steam, apply warm honey on affected parts. Rinse off after 15 minutes.

Gentle Astringents

- ☞ Combine equal of vinegar and water to get an effective astringent.

☞ Tomato juice rubbed over face makes another marvellous astringent off your kitchen shelf.

Saturate cotton wool in pure lemon juice and apply as an astringent.

Mash a small peach and add 4 drops of pure lemon juice and 4 drops of tomato juice to make an astringent lotion.

☞ Grind spinach to extract the juice and use it as an astringent for all skin types especially normal skin.

■

13

Sunburn and Freckles

It has been rightly remarked that "sun can be woman's best friend or her worst enemy". Sun in moderation, lights up your beauty and excess exposure to sun gives your skin the look of old leather.

Sun Burn

Sunlight is excellent for you as it is nature's source of vitamin D. Strong sunlight over prolonged periods are best avoided as it leads to sunburn. Your skin produces melanin which acts as an in-built barrier against ultra violet rays.

Over exposure to sun, causes to UV rays to actually burn up surface skin and penetrate deep into lower cells causing sunburn and other aging problems like lines and wrinkles.

Sunburn is a condition that is better prevented than treated. Sunburn can be a painful affair literally.

Despite your intentions, if you are a victim of sunburn, pamper your skin with

(a) Application of vitamin D ointment.

(b) Use peanut oil, olive oil or lanolin.

(c) Mineral oil can also be used.

Healing properties from your kitchen shelf

☞ Drink plenty of lemon juice before venturing outdoors.

☞ Grate and squeeze cucumber. Spread the seeds and juice over the burn.

☞ Take three small tomatoes and mash well. Add a cup of butter milk. Mix well and apply on skin. Allow to dry for one hour atleast.

This will help to reduce pain and take heat out of skin

- ☞ Cold water compresses together with an additional intake of vitamin A, C and E are recommended for the treatment of sunburn.

  (d) Anti-sunburn lotion

Ingredients : 1 lemon
1 egg white

Method : Add juice of lemon to the white of egg. Whisk briskly, transfer contents to a pan and simmer on low fire till it thickens. Cool it.

Apply to sunburn and do not wash off.

- ☞ Boil lettuce leaves in a cup of boiling water to get a strong infusion which may be applied on sunburn skin.
- ☞ Use whey on your sunburn
- ☞ Yoghurt together with little honey helps to cool and promote healing in sunburnt skin.
- ☞ Combine together a teaspoon of lemon juice with 7-8 drops of milk and gently massage on to skin. Let it soak in before rinsing off with soap and water.

Sun Tan Cream

Ingredients : 2 ounces of lanolin
1 ounce of glycerine
1 ounce of hydrogen peroxide
½ ounce of almond oil

Method : Melt lanolin by using the double boiling method. While still hot, whisk oil and glycerine. Cool completely and add the hydrogen peoxide.

Ingredients : 1 tablespoon of butter milk.

Method : Saturate cotton wool with butter milk and apply. This is a good remedy to remove sun tan.

Ingredients : 1 tablespoon of lemon juice
8 drops of rose water

Method	:	Mix both ingredients, apply and leave on for five to six hours.
Ingredients	:	6 tablespoon of olive oil 6 tablespoon of vineger
Method	:	Combine and apply atleast two hours before your bath.

Freckles

Freckles are spots that appear over bridge of your nose and over your cheeks. Freckles are the outcome of lack of melanin in the skin.

Fading Freckles—The simple method

- ☞ Saturated cotton wood with butter milk and pat on face. Wash off after it has dried.
- ☞ Dip your cotton wool in a solution made by combining one teaspoon of butter milk, one teaspoon of lemon juice and one tablespoon radish juice. Swab face with this and allow to dry before rinsing off.

Apply Anti-freckle Paste

Remove skin of apply and mash it well, apply on freckles everyday.

Oatmeal Paste

Ingredients	:	1 tablespoon oatmeal powder butter milk
Method	:	Add enough butter milk to oatmeal to make a smooth paste.
Application	:	Apply and leave on for twenty minutes and wash off with cold water.

Almond Paste

Ingredients	:	3 almonds 1 egg white 1 teaspoon of lemon juice

Method	:	Grind soaked almonds to a smooth paste. Whisk egg white, add lemon juice and combine. Add to almond paste.
Application	:	Apply on freckles and wash with tepid water. Follow by splashing on cold water.

■

14

How to Gain Youthful Looks

From time immemorial, women loved to posses a smooth and luminous complexion. Preserving youthful complexion eternally has been the secret desire of every woman. The ageing process is inevitable. With the right care you can retain your skin's youthful elasticity and firmness and postpone the advent of lines and wrinkles.

Wrinkles and the loss of natural elasticity results from a damaged mechanism called cross linking. The proteins are bonded together preventing proper functioning of the cellular network.

The epidermal cells slowly loss their capacity for renewal and the dermal cells that produce collagen and elastine slow down their synthesis. The result being dryness, lines and wrinkles on the surface of your skin especially under the eyes, on the forehead and upper lips.

Adverse environmental conditions like over exposure to susceptible to damage while massaging, consumption of alcohol and excessive tobacco smoking.

Anti-ageing powers are now within the grasp of every woman. Cosmetologists have found out effective ways to work against the ageing process. They come in the form of biologically —active creams and liposomes. Use of liposomes bring-forth a marked improvement in resilience and tone of skin.

Skin Rejuvenating

Home made anti-wrinkle creams are safe and effective in producing visible tautening and smoothening benefits. Actively combats wrinkles, lines and bags caused by fatigue and ageing.

Maintain that youthful look by splashing your face with cold water into which powdered nutmeg has been added.

Honey-Caroot Anti-wrinkle Mask

Ingredients	:	1½ tablespoon of honey ½ teaspoon of carrot juice a pinch of soda bi carbonate
Method	:	Combine the honey and juice of carrots.
Application	:	Apply on face. Leave on for twenty minutes. Remove using cotton wool dipped into warm water to which a pinch of bi carbonate of soda has been added.

Cream Mask

Ingredients	:	1 white of an egg 1 tablespoon of cream
Method	:	Combine together to make a paste
Application	:	Apply on face and neck for twenty minutes. Rinse off with tepid water. This mask is said to erase facial lines.

Cornflour Mask

Ingredients	:	1 tablespoon corn flour 1 tablespoon of honey
Method	:	Make a paste with the above ingredients without any lumps.
Application	:	Apply on face and allow it to dry before rinsing off.

Apple Facial Mask

Mash apple and use as a facial mask to postpone wrinkles.

Application	:	Use on face for ten minutes and wash thoroughly with cold water.

Banana mask

Ingredients	:	1 ripe banana 1 tablespoon rose water

Method : Mash banana and mix in rose water

Application : Apply as often as you can. Wash with lukewarm water after thirty minutes. If used regularly it helps to postpone wrinkles.

Mint-Kaolin Mask

Ingredients : 1 egg white
2 tablespoon kaolin
2 tablespoon mint juice

Method : Crush a handful of mint leaves and allow it to steep in water for half an hour. Strain the liquid. Alternatively, you may extract the juice of mint.

Beat the egg white until stiff. Add to the mint extract. Stir in kaolin to make a paste.

Application : Apply this mask all over face and wash it off after fifteen minutes.

Anti-wrinkle Face Pack

Ingredients : 1 teaspoon cucumber juice
1 tablespoon mint juice
1 egg white
½ teaspoon honey
1 teaspoon curd.

Method : Beat egg white until stiff. Blend ingredients thoroughly.

Application : Apply thickly on face. Leave on for fifteen minutes and rinse.

Lanolin Anti-wrinkle Cream

Ingredients : 2 tablespoon lanolin
½ tablespoon honey
2 tablespoon almond oil

Method : Melt lanolin and oil by the double boiling method. Mix in honey.

Application : Apply on face and wash off after fifteen minutes.

Anti-wrinkle Cream

Ingredients : 1 tablespoon of olive oil
1 tablespoon of soda bi carbonate
1 egg

Method : Mix egg and oil briskly.

Application : Apply evenly on face and neck. Allow it to dry. Saturate cotton wool dipped in hot water to which the soda bi carbonate has been added. Gently clean skin surface.

Egg White Facial

Whisk egg white and spread over face to tighten and iron out wrinkles. Rinse off after twenty minutes. You can also use the unbeaten white of an egg. Apply on neck and near eyes.

Anti-wrinkle Lotion

Ingredients : 3 tablespoon witch hazel
1 tablespoon glycerine
1 tablespoon rose water

Method : Combine all the ingredients and blend in a liquidiser for half a minute. Store in a glass jar.

Counteracting Early Wrinkles

- Mashed papaya along with a little cream may be applied regularly.
- Combine together one tablespoon of green gram flour, quarter teaspoon of coconut oil and a generous pinch of turmeric powder. Apply evenly and wash off with cold water after twenty minutes.
- Equal parts of unbeaten white of an egg and glycerine. Mix in quarter teaspoon of rosewater. Stir well and spread on wrinkles. Leave on for twenty minutes and wash with lukewarm water.

■

15

Beauty Aroma Massage

Massage adds glaze to the skin and increases beauty. Regular massage stops premature aging and thus one remains young and energetic for a long time. When problems, diseases and other factors-destroy the natural rhythm of the body and when it becomes dry, ugly, rough, heavy thin etc., certain types of massage can create miracles. If old men and women have 40 days massage every year, they look younger than their age. If one follows the instruction as to food, work, sleep etc., during and after 40 days massage, the old aging signs can be erased.

Massage for beauty starts from the base of the spine. If the spine is not in good shape, the figure of the person will not seem right and one's appearance is one of the most influencing factors in beauty.

After spine, the arms, forearms, palms and fingers are massaged. Then neck, shoulders and lastly the heat and face are massaged. Milk cream, butter and special ubatan for skin texture are applied for massage. If skin of milk or pure cream is applied for massage. If skin of milk or pure cream is applied to any girl or boy of any age group, the effect can be seen within a fortnight. A week before the massage starts for beauty, the diet of the receiver should be fruits, vegetables, nuts, milk, cheese and cream. This diet should be continued not only during the massage but also for a week after the massage course is over.

Massage which consists, chiefly of friction is a doubly valuable aid to beauty. Not only has it the power to improve the condition of the skin and the complexion, but also to give lightness and grace to the whole physical form. Effleurage combined with kneading may form the main part. The effeurage stroke is long and fairly firm and is designed to mould the figure into lines of beauty. To remove stiffness or undue firmness of muscles kneading is necessary which removes all lumpy formation and mould the tissues into graceful lines. Effleurage must be followed by petrissage specially designed to remove imperfection.

The wrists, the ankles, fingers and toes and possibly the neck may be given suitable friction. The friction to the head should designed move the scalp and tapotement with the tips of the fingers is to stimulate the flow of blood.

Delicacy of touch is required not only in treating the face, but also the whole body. The whole series of movements should constitute one unified effort and the general effect should be soothing, pleasant and refreshing.

Women generally use different kinds of cream and talcum powders for beauty. But they have no idea that massage also brings beauty. They have no idea that massage with smooth hand with care, their face will shine like the moon. Kneading, stroking, vibration, clapping etc. may be applied. Knead the cheeks with the palms. For head massage anyone of the following oils can be used:

1. Jeevanthyadi
2. Triphaladi
3. Baladatryadi
4. Neeleebringadi Kuntalakantbi
5. Manjishtadi
6. Eladi
7. Asanaeladi
8. Bhringamalakadi
9. Kumkumadi
10. Malathyadi
11. Brahmi
12. Nasarsha tailam

For the massage of the women's breast Yuvathyadi tailam is advised because that oil not only keeps the breast youth but also brings beauty. For massaging the waist including the sex organ and thigh of women Saubhagya Vardhana tailam may be used. At night while going to bed if the face is massaged with the cream of the milk adding lemon juice and turmeric powder the boils on the face and also small hairs will be disapperared.

For beauty massage about two hours are required. The time is distributed as follow:

Area of massage	**Time of massage**	**Time of relax corpse posture after the are a massage**
1. Spine and Back	15 minutes	10 minutes
2. Hands and Legs	30 minutes	10 minutes
3. Shoulder and Neck	5 minutes	5 minutes
4. Face and Head	30 minutes	15 minutes
Total time for beauty massage	80 minutes	40 minutes

After ubatan is removed from the body a raw milk massage or rose-water bath is adivsed for beauty. In winter sun bath after massage is marvellous. The hair should be washed with Ritha powder, Amala powder, Chickpea flour, yellow clay, goghurt, buttermilk or raw milk as suitable to the subject. During the beauty massage, once in a week more milk and fruit juice diet is essential.

Alcohol, tobacco, meat, fish, egg etc., are strictly prohibited during beauty-massage course.

■

16

Massage According to Dosha Type

Each dosha type requires a different type of massage according to the qualities which are exhibited by the dosha imbalance.

Vata Massage

Because Vatas are already dry, cold, irregular, and rough, they need to have a massage which is oily, warm, smooth and nurturing. Stroking should be firm, but smooth. Abrupt, rough movements can be irritable and disturbing to Vata types. Lots and lots of warm oil should be used. Excess oil can be allowed to sit on the skin (after you've worked on the area) to soak in; Vata bodies will just absorb it. Oil should be allowed to stand and soak into the tissue over the entire abdomen. Keep Vatas warm with sheets, heating pads, even blankets.

Pitta Massage

Pittas are oily, hot, intense and fluid, so they need a massage which is calming and relaxing. They do not need as much oil as Vata types and their oils need to be of a cooling nature. The massage should be deep and varied, and the subject's mind can be kept occupied by using different techniques. Pitta tissues can sometimes be inflamed or irritated, so care should be used in these areas. Too much fast movement can worsen their imbalance; the massage needs to be slow and deliberate without a lot of movement from one area to another. Pittas can become irritable if the therapist is not centred.

Kapha Massage

Kaphas require the most vigorous type of massage to stimulate their sluggish metabolism and lack of fluid movement. Fast, even harsh, movements are appropriate, with as little oil as possible. If the Kapha is really out of balance, increasing amounts of diaphoretic an diuretic essential oils will be helpful. Since you will be using less oil, you can increase the mixture to approximately 75-100 drops of essential oil to four ounces of vegetable oil. During the massage, it's important to draw Kaphas into conversation so they can explore and let go of their own feelings, which they are usually reticent to divulge.

■

17

Skin Care for All Weather

Along with stress and diet, environmental factors are one of the major causes of premature aging. Seasonal and climatic changes not only imbalance the subtle internal energies of the body and mind, but also have an effect externally on the skin. Sun, wind and cold can be particularly damaging unless you take action to counter their effects.

Sun and Skin: The sun has always been a prime offender against the skin, but in recent years its harmful effects have increased as the protective ozone layer has weakened. Solar radiation is a factor in cataracts, cell degeneration and the breakdown of collagen and elastin, which leads to premature aging and wrinkles. It is the leading cause of skin cancer and also increases free radical generation in the skin because it decreases production of antioxidant enzymes. Drugs such as blood pressure pills, diuretics and thorazine and foods and herbs such as artificial sweeteners, carbonated drinks, lemon, lime, carrot, fennel, parsley and bergamot are photo-synthesisers. When ingested and absorbed into the body will cause hyperpigmentation, if the skin is exposed to too much sun. Of course, summer heat aggravates Pitta in general, leading to increased skin sensitivity and increased sebaceous secretions.

In general, sensitive skin types tend to turn red rather than tan in the sun and also develop freckles. Dry and oily skin types both tan easily. Neverthless, nothing ages the skin more quickly than a sunburn, so individuals of every skin type should take precautions to protect themselves from the sun.

Hot Weather Tips for Beautiful Skin

- Warm weather is Pitta season, so adjust your lifestyle and diet to avoid "overheating" the metabolism.

Chlorinated pools, saltwater and sun dehydrate and age the skin, so the body needs extra moisture inside and out all summer long.

- Use a sunscreen with an SPF of 15 to 30 depending upon your skin. If you don't burn easily but do tan easily, use lower SPF. If you burn more easily than you tan, use higher SPF. Try not to use sunscreen unless you are in the sun, since it tends to increase skin sensitivity in general.
- Sesame or neem oil both are excellent natural sunscreens according to Ayurveda.
- Avoid sunbathing. If you want to be in the sun, stay active (do errands, take a walk), but it is better to stay out of the direct sun as much as possible. However, if you do sunbathe, olive and coconut oils are natural tanning agents, since they absorb ultraviolet light and provide even colouring. A daily dose of B-complex vitamins also helps produce an even tan.
- After sunbathing; take a cool bath, adding a few drops rose, sandalwood or vetiver essence to the water. Afterwards, pat the skin dry and when it is still moist, massage all over with your body oil.
- To treat sunburned skin, rub on either crushed cucumber, cucumber juice, aloevera juice, an ice infusion of elderflower and chamomile, or cold buttermilk.

Wind and Skin: Over exposure to dry, cold wind also damages the skin. In addition to their dehydrating effects, cold and wind put pressure on the epidermis, the horny protective top layer of skin which is composed of dead cells. When the cold and pressure are extreme, the dead cells desquamate-they burst-leaving the living, young cells of the derm layer exposed prematurely to the elements. As a result, the unprotected cells become inflamed, causing a characteristic tingling sensation on the skin, a problem that is particularly common among the elderly in the cold season. Too much peeling with acids produces the same result. The best protection against this effect is not face creams, but essential oils.

Cold Weather Tips for Beautiful Skin:

- Cold weather and cool winds aggravate Vata and cause dry skin conditions; so adjust your lifestyle and diet to add warmth, lubrication and moisture.
- Take fewer baths and showers in the cold season to avoid dryness. When you do bathe, add a few drops of essential oil to the water to provide lubrication. Massage with oil before and after showering or bathing.
- Keep the temperature of your home as low as you comfortably can and use a humidifier or keep a bowl of water on your radiators to add moisture to the air.
- Take an occasional steam bath, but avoid saunas, which are dehydrating. Use petroleum jelly, if dryness persists.

■

18

Care for Healthy Hair

Hair is mirror to one's health, whether it is a male or a female; apart from adding to one's personality. But health of hair can be adversely impacted due to mental, emotional and physical disorders, or due to unbalanced diet, pollution factors etc. Moreover, to ensure healthy hair surface should also be massaged.

Oils for Scalp Massage

Avoid using hair dyes, soaps, colourants acid. Instead use conditioners and shampoos that contain jojoba and almond oils. It is said that hot oil treatments permit (essential) oils to soak in easily and also condition the hair. Massage the scalp with warm oil, then wrap the head in a warm towel and, then leave it in the same position for half an hour or so.

Oils for Greasy Hair

Basil, Cedarwood, Chamomile, Cypress, Eucalyptus, Lemon Grass, Rosemary and Sage.

Oils for Normal Hair

Geranium, Lavender, Lemongrass, Rosemary

Oils for Dry hair

Geranium, Lavender, Rose, Sandalwood, Ylang-Ylang.

Method to mix Essential Oils With Base Oils:

You can use any base oil, that suits you the best, out of apricot kernel, sweet almond oil. Evening Primrose, Avocado, jojoba or Sunflower. For massage on one scalp, you can choose upto 3 oils and use 5 drops of each oil to 30 ml base oil.

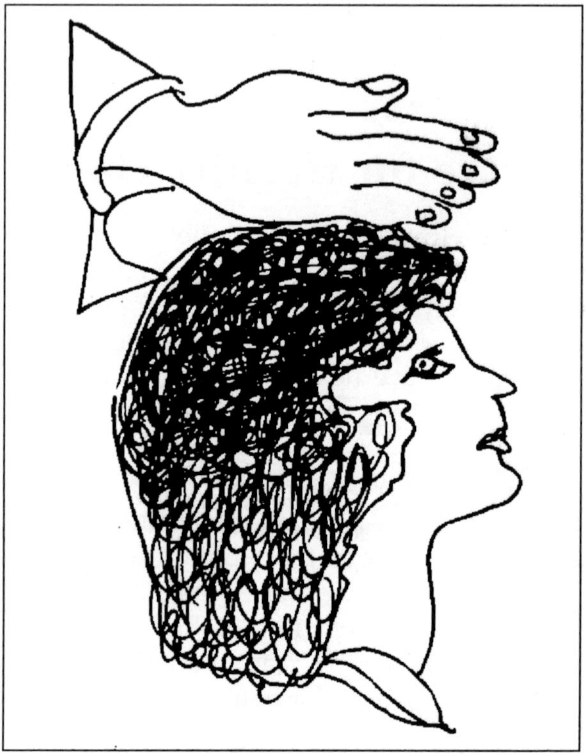

Hair Care

For extra lengthier hair more quantity would be required. Put the bowl, containing blended oil in boiling hot water and then massage into the scalp, whereafter wrap the head with a hot towel and leave it off about 15 minutes and then shampoo.

General Hair Problems

Most of the hair related disorders are dependent on genetic, nutritional, environmental and psychic conditions. When such conditions are massaged, the problem itself will get dispelled and such cases, no medical aid is called for. General hair care can be attended and maintained by proper hygienic and health rules.

Hair Loss

Do not be anxious if hair fall during and after combing. This condition surfaces consequent upon anxiety, stress and hormonal imbalance. So, learn how to relax and avoid tension. Seek guidance and advice of a Tricologist if there is some unusual thinning patch. But you can use blended oil of rosemary and lavender in a base oil for this condition.

Dandruff

Causes of dandruff are many and some of which are poor hair care, bad eating habits, unhealthy life-style, chemical body changes, stress and wrong application of hair products. It is said that hot water baths also precipitate this condition, hence bath with lukewarm water, if weather conditions permit. For rinsing the hair use dandruff shampoos and conditioning rinses which are especially prepared for removal of dandruff. But blended essential oil also serves the purpose. Use cedarwood and lavender oil in a base oil for dry and itchy scalp, and for general treatment use oils of Tea Tree and patchouli. Massage into the scalp with these oils.

Grey Hair

Long standing disease, worry, anxiety, stress, use of hair-dyes for colouring hair, poor diet and irregular eating habits, genetic factors etc. may cause hair to grey. First remove the contributory factor. Use essential oil enhance (like chamomile) to lighten hair and safe for darkening and discolourations.

Scalp Massage

Massage of the scalp is an excellent way to stimulate the scalp, relieve tension and condition hair. If you have small hair, you can massage your scalp yourself but, for long hair, ask another person to do the job for you. Following methods are advised, duly supported by illustrations, for massaging your scalp.

(*a*) Shampoo the hair and towel dry to absord excess water, comb through with a wide tooth comb. Tilt your head and pour some oil in the hairline. Massaging with thumbs on the temple and spread the fingers spread apart over the centre of head.

(*b*) Loosely run fingers and oil over the top of the top of the scalp from front to back lifting hair at the crown. Keeping dipping your fongertips in the treatment oil to spread through the hair while massaging.

(*c*) Massage the head by kneading. Grip and push (with finger pads rather than finger nails) against the scalp. The scalp should gently rotate against the skull. Concentrate on one area at a time with the hands positioned on either side of the scalp.

(*d*) Scalp massage works from front to back, from the forehead, frontal hairline, temples and sides, over the crown of the head to the base of the neck, following the natural flow of blood. If the scalp feel particularly tight then concentrate on areas where the scalp does not want to move. At the base of the skull, press firmly and push the whole scalp up towards the crown to release tension.

(*e*) Pull any extra hair oil through the hair, working out from the roots to the tips. Make sure all the hair is well coiled, and leave towel wrapped for at least 15 minutes before shampooing.

Note—Keeping in mind the condition of your hair, use the most suitable oils (suggested earlier) for better results.

■

19

Care of Body Parts

Essential oils impart pleasure and health benefits, as they absorb quiteably into the warm and damp skin. To prepare body oil choose three bath essential oils (5 drops of each oil) in 2 TBSP (or 30 ml) base oil. In case you wish to prepare larger quantity of body oil, you can use a 3 percent concentration of essential oil to the base oil. Now, after you have prepared a suitable body oil, you can proceed give an after-bath treatment to your body, as suggested hereunder.

Hands and Nails

Hands and nails get affected after daily routine work and if hands are dirty, the dirt will pass on to our stomach with the eaten food. If the filth gets stuck within the nails, it can cause multiple infections. Hence care and hygiene of both hands and nails is pre requisite for our health. If hands are dipped or soaked in water during a bath, the skin gets tender and softer-it will help to clean around the nails and also clip even uneven nails without snagging. Hence the most ideal time for pedicure or manicure is after soaking the hands. For flanky and fragile nails need nourishing and rich treatment, for which they should be rubbed with oil of apricot kernel, Jojoba oil or wheatgerm oil. For moisturising and soothing the hands mix 5 drops each of Lavender, lemon and patchouli oils to 15 ml of sweet almond oil and apply over hands.

Conditioning of Hands and Nails

Hand and nails should be conditioned by way of a simple finger-pulling exercise.

Stretch and spread the fingers straight out. Now massage each finger with blending oils-starting from the tip of the nails to the cuticles and upto the knuckle of each finger.

Feet

Feet are the most neglected part of our body as we take care of them when they are hurt, or pain or ache. Remember, feet have to carry the burden of the entire body and, if feet are tired, aching or hurt, our mobility will be restricted. Moreover, at feet lower extremities also end. While treating your feet, take particular care of beds, soles and toes. Whenever you feel your feet are fatigued or start aching, it is nature's warning signal. While treating your feet after a bath, treat both the feet in entirely and do not adopt a lopsided and casual approach. As skin on and around heels is quite hard, it should be polished hard (around heels and soles) with the help of a punice stone or damp salt. If you want to stimulate blood circulation and also relax your tired feet, you should bend one knee (while in the bath) grip the toes first and thereafter massage in an upward direction-starting from the toes and then going upwards to heels and finally to calves. Body oil should be massaged into the feet after you have taken a bath, shower or peicure.

Add 3 drops each of lavender and cypress oils to a basin full of water (so as to gain deidrising and soothing effect) and bathe your feet. If you have chiblains, mix 3 drops of geranium and one drop each of rosemary and lavender oils to 1 TBSP of base oil of sweet almond and then massage the affected parts.

Massage in between the toes (after a bath) and then move around the tougher skin and heel areas, in order to soften the feet. In order to stimulate blood circulation to each hook and corner of the feet, finish with sweeping movements all over the area.

Elbows

Elbows are generally neglected during and after bath. But such a neglect can result in build up of hard protective layers of grey and unsightly skin. Certain persons have tougher and rough skin around the elbow. But the problem can be easily encountered by application of sweet almond oil and fine oatmeal, for which 3 TBSP each of sweet almond oil and fine oatmeal should be mixed to prepare a paste, add yoghurt or milk to it. This paste should be rubbed over the elbows and any grey spot and goosey areas of skin around the upper arms. If arms are flabby add to the past 6 drops of fennel oil also. Another cheaper and traditional method to cut a lemon into 2 pieces, squeeze out the juice and then rub the elbow in the hollow of the lemon. Some persons mix lemon juice and glycerine also for the same purpose, adding also a few drops of sweet oil of almond. Oil is being applied to the arms with smooth upward strokes. You should concentrate more on the elbows and upper arms where the skin is often found to be drier and rougher.

Applying body oil to neck, shoulders and back

As it is quite difficult to reach the areas of neck, shoulders and back either, during or after a bath, these remain neglected, even though these area and skin around them should be nourished to release tension. Massage the said areas with a suitable body oil as smoothly as possible. It is better to seek another person's help in this regard.

■

20

Massage of Legs/Hand

This process consists of two methods, viz Effleurage and leg stretching (The term 'effleurage' means that when a masseur passes his/her hands continuously and rhythemically over a person's skin in one direction only, with the aim of increasing the flow of blood in that direction and aiding the dispersal of any swelling due to edema'—*A.L. Harrison*)

Effleurage

To begin with apply oil to both the legs using effleurage movement working from the ankles upwards, as in the same manner as detailed in the case of massage bck of the legs. In order to ensure even distribution of oil, repeat the sequence of effleurage several times.

Leg Stretch

Support the leg at the ankle and behind the knee, bend the leg up and place the same in line with the shoulder. Clasp your hands around the back of the knee and ask your partner to inhale deeply, then pull the calf muscle toward you. Hold the calf muscle for a slow count of 3. When your partner breathes out, release your pull on the calf muscles.

Above detailed movement should be repeated 3 times, after which let the leg be laid down. Then, repeat the stretch on the other leg also.

Effleurage on Hands and Arms

(a) Be seated to the side of your partner and, then slightly move one arm away from her. Now apply oil from just above the wrist, upto the shoulder and round.

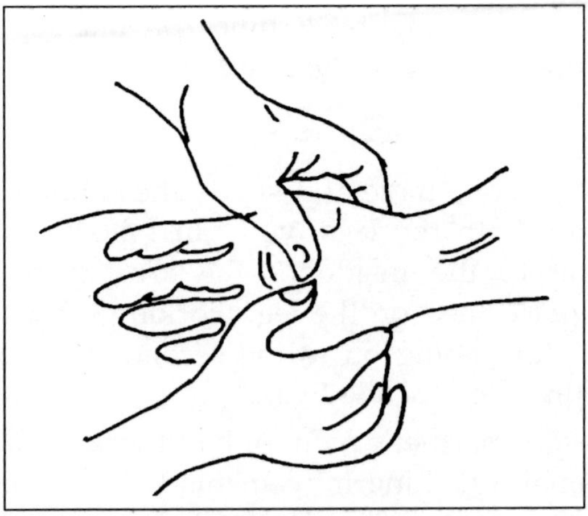

Palm Massage

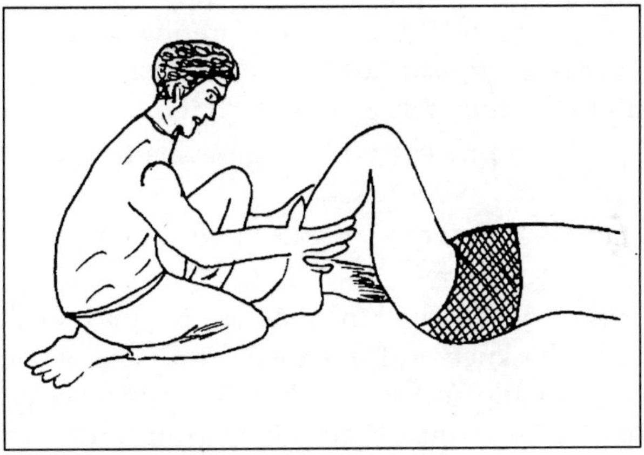

Leg Massage

(b) Now your first arm should come off the arm, while the other hand will start (movement) at the wrist and sweep uptoward the gland that is seated in the joint of elbow.

(c) Now the first hand should cross the second hand as it reaches the elbow and sweeps again from wrist to the shoulder.

Repeat this movement 6-7 times on one leg and, then, repeat the same process on the other leg also.

Hand Massage

[**Note**—When you have finished the above described movements on both the legs, you can follow the effleurage with flushing to the inside of the arm, using the same movements performed on the leg, working from the wrist to the elbow. Before going on to the second arm, massage the hand of the first are.—**Make Evans**.]

(a) Rest your partner's palm of hand over your palm, and use small brushing movements with the help of your thumbs so as to work upward between the joints of the fingers towards the wrist.

(b) Pulling back to the fingers, gently massage the joint between your thumb and forefinger as you draw towards the tips of fingers. Then finish up with a slight pull to the finger so as to stretch it out.

(c) Repeat the process with finger, finally finishing with the thumb.

Repeat the identical movements on the other hand and arm also.

When you have finished the massage the partner should be covered upto the knee and make sure that she is completely relaxed, comfortable and warm. Now let her relax or rest for 5-15 minutes. After requisite rest, help your partner in sitting up rather carefully and after a glassful of water is required.

■

21

Baby Massage

Massage is a marvellous way to enhance the natural bounding between the mother and the (new born) baby as touch is a natural way to establish contact between both. All babies instantly respond to cuddling and caressing. You must have noticed how a baby tightly curls its hands and feet when touched. Since I have given reasonably detailed account of massage with blending of essential oils with carrier oils in the case of elders but in the case of babies, no essential oil is used, but only light vegetable oils, like sweet almond, sunflower and baby oil or olive oil are used.

Advantages and Significant points about Massage

- Unless okayed by an aromatherapist, no essential oil should be added to the massage oil.
- Do not expose baby's tender skin to strong or biting cold, cold winds and snow fall.
- Warm your hands before the massage. It is still better if oil is also slightly warmed.
- Gently stroke baby's tender body and do not exert any pressure.
- Do not massage when the baby is weeping or is ill or when he resists any type of touch even.
- Room should be warm, quiet and without any draughts.
- Massage relieves babies colic, alleviates wind, improves digestion, cures coughs, and colds etc.
- Keep movements gentle and smooth flowing.
- Massage builds up general resistance of body.

☞ Do not apply any oil to baby's face and eyes.

☞ Do not massage immediately before, during or after a feed.

Make sure that massage helps your baby to feel lighter and better and that no discomfort or agitation is caused to it. If the baby weeps or cries during the massage, it means the massage area is either painful or too sensitive. In such a situation stop massaging. You may restart when the baby feels comfortable.

Proceed as Follows

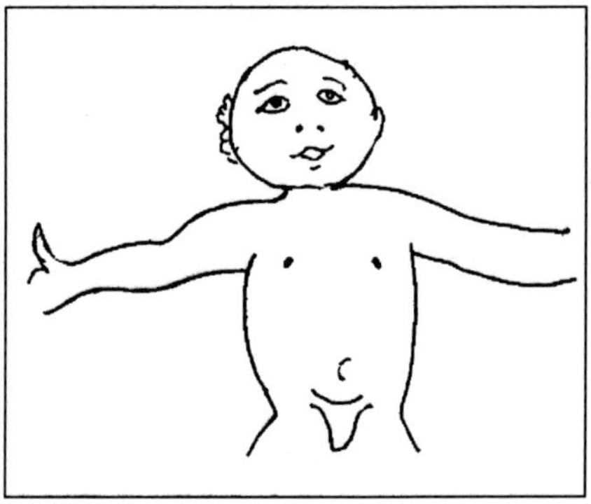

Take a large sized towel and spread half portion there of on your legs or on laps and the other half under the baby's back but ensure there are no wrinkles or folds. Lay the baby on its back, or lay him in the position that makes him feel comfortable. Apply some oil to your palms and, then, apply gently and softly over the frontal portion of his body. Use oil of sweet almond 5 ml. Ensure that your hands are warm, room is also warm and quiet, and also there are no draughts. You can massage baby's body either before the bath or after the bath, but ideal time should preferably is said to be after the bath.

Frontal Massage of the Baby

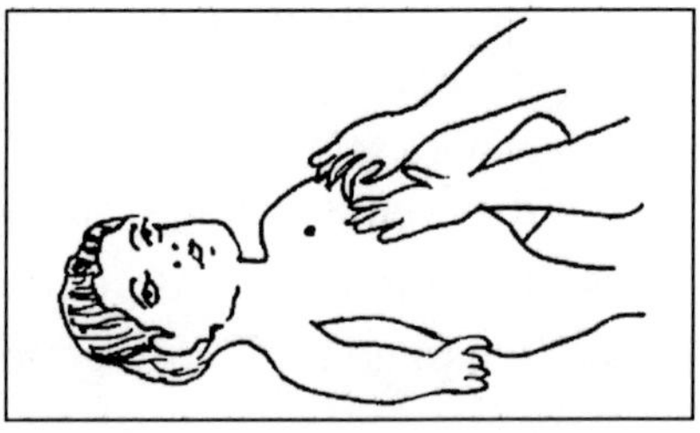

(a) Gently and slowly apply a little quantity of the oil over its front of the body, from shoulders to feet, but avoid the face. Now lightly stroke down the

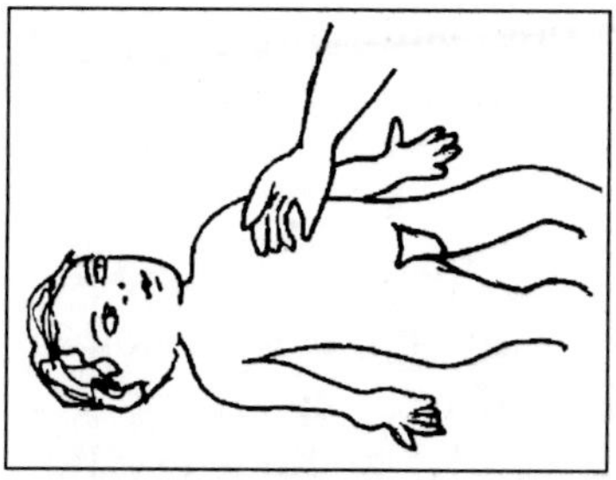

chest and abdomen using the tips of your fingers. By your light and delightful strokes, you can calm your baby at any time. Remember, touch of hands in the body will cheer up the baby and he will show his happiness through light laughter or innocent smile. Let his legs be kept in a straight line but if he curls up his legs, let him do so. It is a sign that he is enjoying and releasing the movements.

(b) Keep the pressure very light, move both your hands smoothly in continuous and circular strokes over the abdomen, working up the baby's right side across and down his body's left side. Keep your movements continuous by lifting your left hand when your arms cross. Now repeat such circular movements many a time.

Left Side

(c) If your baby lets you, gently stretch out both the arms to the sides, spreading hands and fingers. Then gently squeeze out along the arms and, with light and circular thumb movements massage his palms and wrists. Before you finish your movements, do not forget to stretch out his each finger with a light pull.

(d) Now move on to legs and feet, but work out only on one leg at a time. Supporting baby's leg with both of your hands gently squeeze and release fleshy part of his thigh.

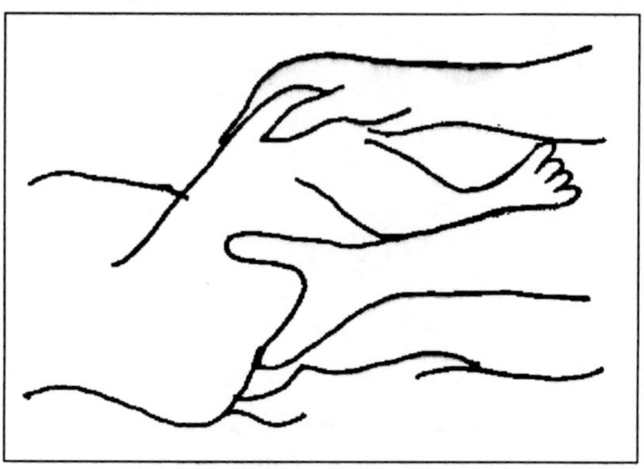

Thereafter, support the leg with one hand and stroke the leg, from knee to the thigh and back down again.

Right Side

Now move your supporting hand down to behind the ankle. Then gently smooth palm of your hand over top of baby's foot-that is from toe to ankle and back again. As you reach the toes, stretch each toe very gently, without exerting any force/pressure.

The same steps should be repeated 4-5 times on baby's other leg also.

Baby's Back side Massage

(a) Now turn the baby over onto the front. Then start to stroke up his entire back side so that applied oil is evenly distributed to the whole of the back side. After applying the oil evenly over his back side, work up your strokes around baby's side also, and then up the legs, back and out over the arms. If you massage his back side, as suggested, it will have very calming impact on the baby's spinal nerves, because soothing effect always cheers the baby up.

(b) To stimulate the blood circulation, gently knead and squeez its buttocks. For this you should make a loose fist and rotate over the baby's buttocks in circular movements.

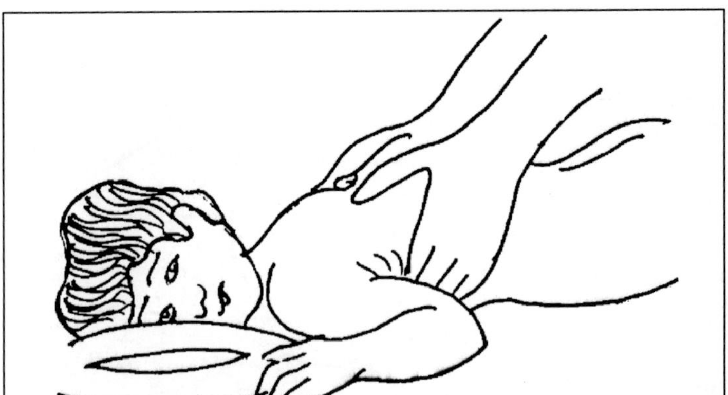

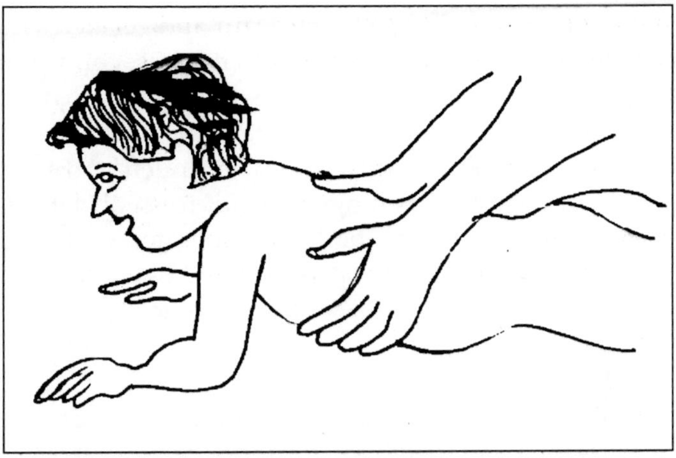

(c) Now gently stroke up one side of the back to the shoulders and down again. Repeat the suggested movements on the other side of the back also.

(d) Now bring both of your hand's around the scetes of your body and, then, using your thumbs, massage gently up the back to the base of the neck. You should also massage baby's shoulders with the help of thumbs.

(e) Finally, before you finish up, repeat the feather strokes that were used at the beginning of the massage, by working all over the back, from neck to buttocks.

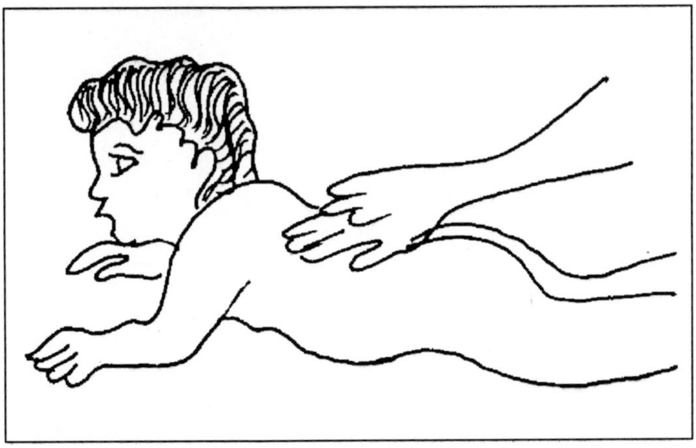

See how a baby feels happy, cheerful and relaxed when its mother holds it in her hands, looks into its eyes, communicates with the baby in a motherly affectionate and caressing mood. There is also a sort of indirect exercise for the baby. It is simply a cheerful reaction of affirmity, affection, touch and nearness. When the infant laughs, its lungs expand, fresh air lets in, skin smoothen, eyes sparkle and body reverberates with renewed energy. If you cling her to your breast, she will feel still reassured, secure and filled up with confidence.

Massage For Everyone

Remember how as a child if you bumped your head (or anywhere else) a wise adult would kindly rub it better? Or that if any part of your body aches now it's instinctive to put your hand there?

Very simply, this how massage works. Touch is both healing and comforting and, what's more, we can all enjoy the pleasures of it—both giving and receiving. massage is beneficial to us in several different ways and:

- ☞ Improves blood circulation
- ☞ Calms the nervous system
- ☞ Stimulates skin function
- ☞ Improves muscle tone
- ☞ Eases aches and pains in muscles and joints

And it feels marvellous!

■

22

Help for Stretch Marks

Stretch marks are actually little tears in the tissue beneath the skin surface, and they show up first as red or purplish marks which fade to a silvery white scar. They are caused by the skin stretching as your weight increases, and you are more prone to them during pregnancy when your weight gain is rapid. Some skins have a better capacity to stretch than others, so pregnancy doesn't necessarily mean you'll get stretch marks. Although I don't believe that by applying oils and lotions you can prevent stretch marks (the damage occurs quite deep in the skin), you can help to keep your skin elastic and supple. Also, by using aromatherapy oils, you can minimise the scarring and speed up the skin's healing process.

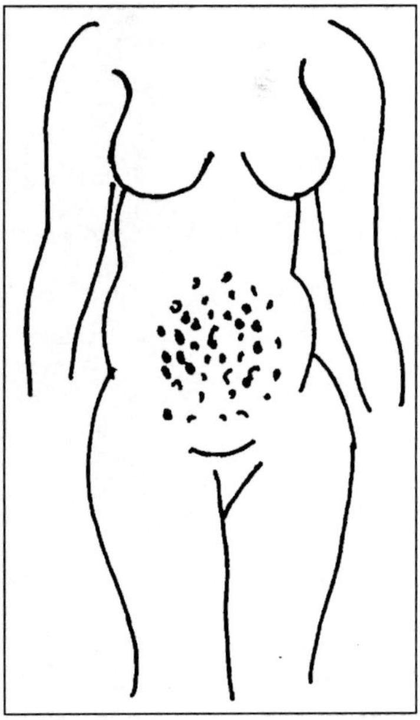

Aromatherapy Strech Mark Oil

Add three drops of frankincense and three drops of tangerine oil to a carrier blend of 2 fl oz (50 ml) of avocado oil and 2 fl oz (50 ml) of wheatgerm oil. Frankincense has a rejuvenating effect on your skin and tangerine oil is rich in Vitamin C and helps to maintain your skin's elasticity.

I recommend you start using this blend from the beginning of your pregnancy, paying special attention to your breasts, tummy, hips and thighs. Massage it gently into all those areas at least once a day. A good time to do this is at night, after your bath, when your skin is soft.

You may also like to try the following breast massage, as your breasts will increase in size during pregnancy and are therefore prone to stretch marks and tissue damage.

Breast Massage

Apply the stretch mark oil to your breasts.

1. Gently work around each breast in a circular movement with your whole hand. Repeat five or six times.
2. Now, place the heel of each hand on either side of one breast and gently stroke in towards the nipple. Repeat five or six times.
3. Next, move your hands to the top and underside of the breast and again stroke into the nipple. Repeat five or six times.
4. Gently stretch each nipple with your fingertips.
5. Repeat step 1.

■

23

Benefits of Massage

Benefits of massage are mentioned in the ancient book of Ayurveda. They are:

1. Jarahar (Remover of old age)

Daily massage to the spine, feet (soles) and heat with Almond oil increases virility and semen. The body is made of seven ingredients, such as:

(a) Rasa (hormones, fluids, lymph)
(b) Rakta (blood)
(c) Mamsa (flesh)
(d) Medha (tendons of nerves)
(e) Asthi (bones, teeth, nails)
(f) Majja (marrow)
(g) Shukra (semen)

Massage provides energy to all the seven ingredients and oil age symptoms approach late.

2. Shramahar (Remover of fatigue)

By physical and mental strain one feels fat gue. It affects the muscles and causes tension. Rubbing, patting and squeezing muscles gently remove fatigue.

3. Vatahar (Remover of humour of wind)

Rheumatism is one of the ailment caused by wind. Daily massage with Maha Narayana taila or other such Ayurvedic oils help to remove the troubles created by wind or gases.

4. Darsanakar (Increases sight)

Regular massage improves sight and keeps blindness and other diseases of eyes away. Feet massage especially under the big toe and also massage of spine, neck and head will remove eye troubles and improve vision.

5. Pushtikar (Strengthener)

By rubbing, pressing, kneading etc. the circulation of vital life fluids increases and makes the body strong.

6. Ayuṣhkar (Supplier of longevity)

By massage the longevity increases.

7. Swapnakar (That brings sleep)

Massage induces sleep. Head and feet massage with pumpkin seed oil before going to bed gets the patient sleep.

8. Twakdhritakar (Skin strengthener)

Massage makes the skin smooth, shining and strong. Dryness is the sign of disturbed wind element in the body.

Some times dryness comes by meditation, mental work, anxieties and worries. The people in cold regions get dry skin facing the chilled air.

9. Klesha Sahatwa (Tolerate troubles)

Resistance against disease and disharmony increases by massage because it excites production of antibodies and strengthen the above mentioned seven ingredients. The anti bodies give more resistance to disease and the strength of seven terms gives tolerance.

10. Abhighat Sahatwa (Tolerate injuries)

One who gets massage regularly recovers injuries more quickly than others who do not get massage.

11. Kapha-Vata Nirodhaka: (Protector from the troubles of mucous and wind)

Regular massage protects from the trouble of mucous and wind.

12. Mrija Varna baiaprada (Giver of colour and strength to skin)

By massage the colour and the texture of the skin improves and hence it gets more strength. So Ayurvedic massage is highly praised by using oils.

■

24

How to Take a Bath

A bath is a daily ritual, but few people understand its purpose or importance. That is why most of us merely throw water over our heads and the bodies and think that we have done our duty. Throwing water over the body is beneficial but it is not what a bath is.

The twin purposes of a bath are: cleanliness and reactivating the circulation of the blood by the bringing sensation that cold water produces as it comes into contact with the skin. The first purpose, i.e. cleanliness can be better served by hot water. The skin of the body has millions of pores through which the skin breathes as we do through our lungs. If the pores are clogged, the lungs are overworked. Overwork may lead to fatigue or exhaustion of the lungs, and then, closed pores do not pass any perspiration which the skin breathes or we do through our lungs. And then, closed pores do not pass any perspiration which is a must to clear the blood of morbid humours. Closed pores are a danger to the general health of human beings.

Cold water is also a cleansing agent, but it cannot deal with the grease and dirt infesting the pores of the skin. Hot water mixed with lemon juice is the best cleansing agent for the skin. Or better still, take a lemon and roast it lightly over a fire. Then cut it into two parts, dip a part in hot water and rub it over your skin. This will cleanse your skin as no soap can do. But a hot bath should not be taken daily. It generally bring weakness and slows down the digestive processes. Once or twice a weak is enough if you have to take hot bath. The temperature of the water should not be more than one or two degree above body temperature.

A hot bath before retiring for the night is the best for your health. It helps you to sleep better and if you cover your body after a hot bath, it will save you from the danger of exposure. A bath hot or cold should be taken one hour before meals or three hours after it.

Really hot water for a bath has its own advantages but it should be used sparingly. If you are suffering from a cold, take a hot bath, cover yourself with woollens and get into bed. It will drive away the cold. A really hot bath when you are tired acts as a tonic: it drives away fatigue as nothing else does.

A bath with hot water has its uses, but a daily bath should be with cold water. When the skin is cooled by the cold water, blood rushes to warm it up. The circulation of the blood is activated and the blood is also cleansed of many impurities. A slowed down circulation is a prelude to old age. A cold bath is, therefore, instrumental in keeping us young.

The best way to start a bath is to rub the whole of your body with your palms or with a rough towel. Start with your scalp, forehead, face and the neck. Then go on to your wrists and then to the shoulders through the arms. Afterwards nib your chest, the armpits and abdomen and the back. The feet should be the 1st to receive attention. Keep your feet straight when you rub them. Start from the feet and come upto the thighs. In the begining, rub gently but later increase the pressure.

After the vigorous rubbing, take a cold bath. Wipe your body with a towel. Start with the head and then dry up the whole body. You will feel a peculiar kind of pleasure when you rub your body after a bath. For weak persons a rubbing can do the job of exercise.

If this method of taking a bath is adopted, there will not be any danger of any skin eruptions or itch. The face will be free of pimples and other blemishes which mar its beauty. The skin will acquire a healthy glow and if it is rough and leathery, it will become pink and soft. You will have the feeling as if you have been having an oil massage.

■

25

Different Baths

Here you will find variety of baths with their procedures and benefits.

Neutral Bath

The neutral bath, sometimes called the continuous bath, is a non-thermic hydrotherapy of great value. It consists of whole body immersion in water approximately 92 to 97oF.

Indications: Insomnia, nervous exhaustion, anxiety, depression

Contra-indications: Diabetes, arteriosclerosis, fever, acute hypertension, chronic pain, toxemia of pregnancy, peripheral edema, cardiac weakness, eczema or other skin condition aggravated by water.

Equipment: Full-size bathtub, bath thermometer, towels, pillow, sheet.

Procedure: Fill full-size bathtub with water of neutral temperature.

Make client comfortable with pillow or rolled towel for neck support; adjust water to temperature neutral to client. Client should feel somewhere between "comfortably warm" and neither warm nor cold. This is a better guide that the thermometer, although the actual temperature also should be monitored. Cover and exposed parts (e.g. knees) with towels or cover whole tub with sheet. Lighting should be dim. Add water, as necessary, to maintain neutral temperature. Cool water a few degrees at the end of the treatment and assist client out of tub. Dry quickly but gently without friction, which would be too stimulating for a curative treatment. Let client rest for half an hour.

Duration: Fifteen minutes to one hour for insomnia.

Hot Tub Bath

The hot bath treatment consists of full immersion in water approximately 104°F. The entire body, with the exception of the head, is immersed in water. While immersed, the body can not control its temperature by sweating; although the client's body can release some heat through the head. The body temperature rises and the detoxification process begins.

Indications: Poor circulation, pain, muscle stiffness ad general fatigue, congestion of internal organs.

Contra-indications: Heart disease; diabetes; diseases of malignant origin such as acute cancer, acute swelling and wounds; vascular disorders; high blood pressure.

Procedure: Fill tub two-thirds full of hot water. The temperature should be 104°F. Assist client into tub. Cover exposed body parts with a towel or cover tub with a sheet or light blanket. Keep head cool with a cold compress. Check pulse regularly. Do not let pulse exceed eighty beats per minute.

Assist client from tub. Follow the bath with an alcohol rub or a cool sponge bath. Dry thoroughly and keep client warm. Let client rest one hour after treatment.

Duration: One to twenty minutes.

Cold Tub Bath

The cold tub bath is a powerful stimulant. Use only with well conditioned clients. Treatment consists of full immersion in water approximately 75°F.

Indications: Gradual vascular conditioning, common cold in an otherwise healthy person, following a strong heat treatment, fever.

Contra-indications: Weakness from an infection, cardiac disease, chilliness (heat first), menstruation, allergy to cold, severe diabetes.

Procedure: Fill the tub two-thirds full with water. The temperature should be about 75°F. Assist client into tub. Rub client vigorously with bath mitten. Assist client from tub. Dry client thoroughly.

Duration: Fifteen seconds to thirty seconds.

Whirlpool Bath

The whirlpool bath combines the thermal stimulus of the water with further mechanical stimuli. One way in which this occurs is with the aid of a rotating propeller, which moves the water. In addition, warm air is injected into the water through a small nozzle. Depending on its size, the whirlpool bath can be used either as a partial bath for the lower legs or the arms, or as a full bath for the entire body. The whirlpool bath should not be compared to the underwater massage, as the mechanical component is weaker. One of the outstanding therapeutic uses of the whirlpool is to relieve muscle soreness and fatigue. This is the reason many athletes and dancers purchase portable whirlpools for their baths, or go swimming in a pool with such whirlpool action. Whirlpool baths are helpful in anti-pain therapy.

Indications: Injuries, rheumatic disabilities, including rheumatic muscle and joint diorders, muscle soreness, fatigue, raynaud's disease, tennis elbow, knee joint problems, swollen joints of arthritis, to improve the circulation of paraplegic and polio victims. Whirlpool therapy can help with circulation problems and it is a well-known aid in relieving chronic pain and the phantom pain that occurs after amputations. It will also help to heal skin sores and infected wounds, reduce the swelling of chronic edema (tissue swelling), help reduce the pain of minor frostbite, ease scar tissue from burns, and help with weak and painful feet. Many physiotherapists prepare their clients for therapy massage by first giving them a stimulating and relaxing whirlpool bath.

Contra-indications: Sensitive to very hot water, diabetes, varicose veins, advanced arteriosclerosis or any advanced vascular limb problem.

Procedure: Assist client into tub. Start the whirlpool bath at a neutral temperature, and raise to the tolerance of the client. Allow client to relax in tub. Assist client from tub. If you are following the whirlpool with a massage, wrap the entire body so that it stays completely warm.

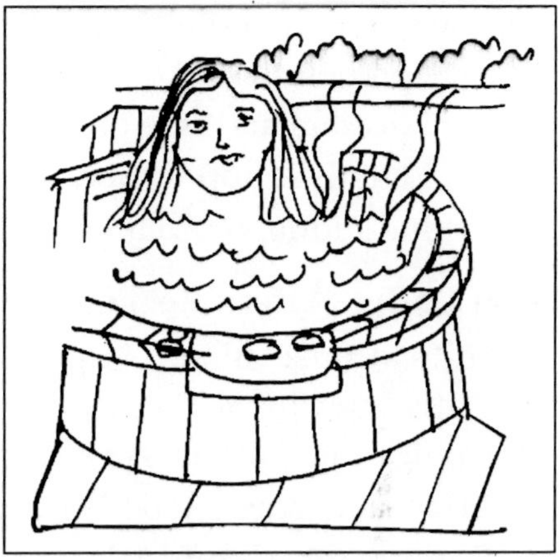

Whilrpool Bath

Duration: Fifteen to forty-five minutes, depending on the purpose for which it is being used.

The Kneipp Baths

In the Kneipp treatments, baths are given as:

- Arm bath
- Foot bath
- Hip bath
- Half bath
- Three-quarter bath
- Full bath

These baths may be taken (temperature):

- Cold 32-65°F
- Cool 66-71°F
- Lukewarm 72-82°F
- Intermediate 83-95°F
- Warm 96-100°F
- Hot 101-105°F

Warm baths may be taken with herbal additives such as balm mint, chamomile, lavender, meadow flower or pine needle.

The strength of the stimulus is determined by:

- Temperature
- Location and size of area
- Length of application
- Individual pretreatment disposition

Arm Bath—Alternate Temperature

Indications: Blood circulation problems, high blood pressure, bronchitis.

Contra-indications: Angina pectoris, heart ailments.

Effects: Increases blood circulation.

Equipment: Comfortable chair, two arm baths or wash basins.

Procedure: Have client seated comfortably.

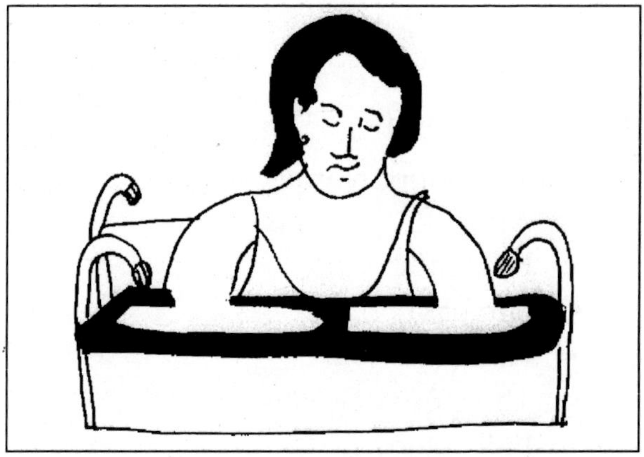

Arm Bath—Alternative Temperature

Fill one arm bath with warm water, 96 to 100°F. Fill another arm bath with cold water, 65°F. Dip both arms in the warm water, up to the middle of the upper arm. Repeat the procedure in cold water. Wipe off the arms with hands. Do not towel dry. Exercise arms until warm. One hour of bed rest is recommended.

Duration: 1. Five minutes warm water. 2. Ten seconds cold water. 3. Five minutes warm water. 4. Ten seconds cold water.

Herbal Bath

Additives: In warm water only: Balm mint, chamomile, lavender, meadow flower, pine needle, rosemary.

Arm Bath—Increasing Temperature

Indications: Angina pectoris, high blood pressure, cardiovascular insufficiency, headache, asthma, bronchitis, local non-inflammatory rheumatism.

Contra-indications: Lymph blockage, lymph edema of the arms, varicose veins.

Effects: Vasodilatation, improves blood circulation.

Equipment: Comfortable chair, arm bath or wash basin.

Procedure: Have client seated comfortably. Fill the arm bath with warm water, 83 to 95°F. Dip both arms in arm bath, up to middle of upper arm. Raise the temperature of water gradually to 105°F. (This should take fifteen to twenty minutes). Towel dry arms, fifteen to thirty minutes. Bed rest is recommended.

Duration: Fifteen to twenty minutes.

Herbal Bath

Additives: In warm water only: Balm mint, chamomile, lavender, meadow flower, pine needle, rosemary.

Foot Bath—Cold Temperature

Indications: Venous circulatory disorders, tired feet.

Contra-indications: Acute bladder/kidney infections, oversensitivity to cold, female pelvic disorders, coronary deficiencies.

Effects: Stimulates metabolism, alleviates insomnia, sleep inducing in the evening, influences venous blood flow return, increases blood circulation.

Equipment: Foot bathtub or large bucket.

Procedure: Fill the footbath with cold water, 54°F. With the water as cold as client can tolerate. Instruct client to dip both feet into footbath. The client can sit in a chair or stand for this procedure, whichever is most comfortable. Wipe water off feet with hands. Do not towel dry. To keep feet warm, leg exercises or bed rest should follow the treatment.

Duration: Fifteen seconds to one minute.

Foot Bath—Warm Temperature

Indications: Arterial circulation disorders, chronic infection (e.g., nose, throat, pharyngeal), weak immune system, chronic constipation, chronic cold feet, preparation for pedicure, after acute phase of ankle/foot contusion.

Contra-indications: Varicose veins, hypertension.

Effects: Increases blood circulation, alleviates insomnia, soothes, relaxes.

Equipment: Foot bathtub or large bucket.

Procedure: Fill the footbath with warm water, 97 to 100°F. Instruct the client to dip both feet in the water. Towel dry feet. Follow with bed rest for at least thirty minutes.

Duration: Ten to fifteen minutes.

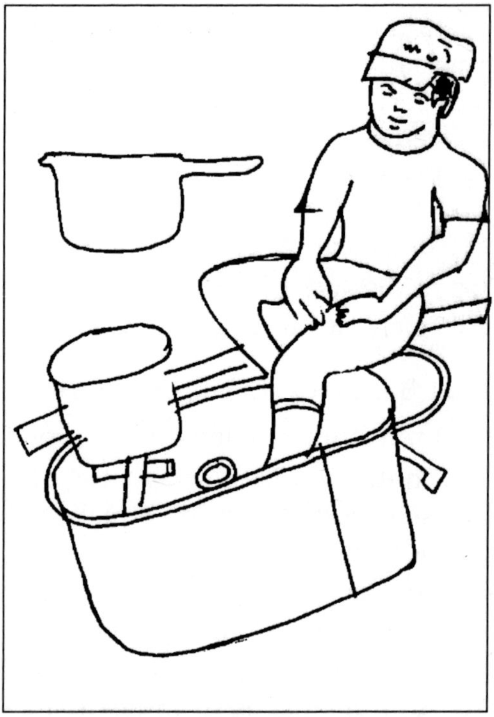

Foot Bath

Herbal Bath

Additives: Balm mint, chamomile, lavender, meadow flower, pine needle, rosemary.

Foot Bath—Alternate Temperature

Indications: Chronic cold feet, low blood pressure, insomnia.

Contra-indications: Varicose veins.

Effects: Increases effectiveness of the body's heat regulatory system, improves blood circulation, stabilises the nervous system.

Equipment: Two foot bathtubs or two large buckets.

Procedure: Fill one bath with warm water, 97 to 100°F and one bath with cold water, as cold as the client can tolerate. Instruct the client to put both feet in the warm water for five minutes, then into the cold water for ten to fifteen seconds. Repeat the procedure. Wipe feet with hands. Do not towel dry. Exercise legs until warm or follow with bed rest for one hour.

Duration: 1. Five minutes warm water. 2. Ten to fifteen seconds cold water. 3. Five minutes warm water. 4. Ten to fifteen seconds cold water.

Herbal Bath

Additives: For warm water only: Balm mint, chamomile, lavender, meadow flower, pine needle, rosemary.

Foot Bath—Increasing Temperature

Indications: Acute and chronic bladder/kidney infections, begining colds (symptoms like sneezing, chills, feeling weak and tired), cold feet, vascular headache, non-inflammatory problems, leg cramps, menstrual problems.

Contra-indications: Varicose veins, phlebitis (blood clots), heart problems, minor circulatory problems.

Effects: Increases blood circulation to organs (i.e., pelvic areas). Increases body temperature in feet immediately.

Equipment: Foot bathtub or large bucket.

Procedure: Fill the footbath with warm water 83 to 95°F. Gradually raise water temperature to 101 to 103°F. (This should take fifteen to twenty minutes.) Towel dry feet. Follow with bed rest for at least fifteen to thirty minutes.

Duration: Fifteen to twenty minutes.

Herbal Bath

Additives: Balm mint, chamomile, lavender, meadow flower, pine needle, rosemary.

Mineral, Herbal, and Essential Oil Baths

There are many herbal and pharmaceutical substances that can be added to baths to produce special effects.

Water by itself has a remarkable, almost magical ability to alter the body state. Depending on the specific need, water will decrease or increase muscle tone, reduce pain, or generate energy. The addition of certain herbal and pharmaceutical substances to the water is a twin present to the body. Some herbs soothe, others sedate or stimulate, and others soften the skin. Most important is the ability of some substances to hasten perspiration or to stimulate release of stored toxins from within the body. This ability helps to overcome many symptoms and can improve a chronic condition.

Fango (Mud) Salicyl Powder Bath

This bath is the ultimate. It is the favourite fragrant mud bath in European Spa Kur therapy centres. Its soothing effects are due to the combination of the analgesic properties of the volcanic ash powder (fango) and the pine needle essential oil.

Indications: Rheumatism in muscles and joints, sciatica, neuritis, degenerative non-inflammatory joint arthrosis, lumbago.

Effects: Stimulates circulation, replaces minerals, exfoliates the skin.

Equipment: Bathtub, shower, towels, fango (mud) salicyl powder (ingredients: salicyl powder, natrium humat, pine needle extract).

Procedure: Dissolve the powder in hot water, Assist client into bath, and allow to soak for ten to twenty minutes. Assist client from bath and into a cool shower. Wrap client in warm blanket and allow to rest.

Whey (High Protein Milk Serum) Bath

Whey is a high-protein milk serum. Liquid cow's milk has about 6.25 percent protein; of that, 80 percent is contained in the whey. Traditionally, the term whey protein describes those milk proteins that remain after the cheese-making process uses up the casein molecules. In bygone days, whey was fed to young livestock on the farm because of its nutritional value.

Whey is a complete protein containing all the essential and non-essential amino acids found in nature. Long ago Hippocrates promoted the health and beauty benefits of whey. It was also very popular during the Renaissance. Today it is Europe's foremost skin care bath product.

It is also called "lacto-med-derm bath" (lacto meaning produced from milk, med meaning medically tested, and derm for skin friendly).

Indications: Particularly useful for aging and dry skin, neurodermatitis, psoriasis, acne, eczema, baby rash, fungus, sunburn, and other skin ailments.

Equipment: Bathtub, towel, washcloth, whey bath powder (ingredients: lactose, milk fat, milk protein, graham salt, magnesium carbonate, wintergreen essential oil).

Procedure for bath: Client should be encouraged to bathe in the whey bath at least three times per week. Fill tub two-thirds full with warm water, 95°F. Assist client into bath. Allow client to soak ten to twenty minutes.

Procedure for mask: The whey powder can also be used as a mask on the face, hands, and feet. Assure powder to a wet, warm washcloth. Apply washcloth to client's skin (face, hands, and/or feet). Remove after ten to fifteen minutes.

Mud Natrium Powder Bath

The fango (mud) natrium powder bath, used in spas worldwide, is a mineral-rich volcanic ash extract. This ancient beauty ritual is effective for removing impurities and smoothing the texture of the skin so it can readily absorb moisture and minerals. Fango (mud) natrium powder is biologically pure, bacteria free, unscented and fully dissolves in bath water. It will not stain the tub or body.

Indications: Tired muscles

Effects: Will detoxify and revitalise the body.

Equipment: Bathtub, shower, towels, fango (mud) natrium powder (ingredients: 100 percent unscented natrium humat volcanic ash extract)

Procedure: Fill bathtub two-thirds full. Dissolve powder into bath. Assist client into tub and allow to soak for ten to twenty minutes. For a real spa kur treatment, let the client shower with cool or cold water after the bath. Client should then rest, while warmly wrapped, for ten to twenty minutes.

Mustard Powder Bath

The great healing virtues of mustard have been extolled by numerous civilisation for thousands of years. The Greeks, including Hippocrates, the Romans, the early American settlers, and Native American all used mustard for medicinal purposes. The most universally known use of mustard is in a mustard plaster, recommended for common congestions of the lung. Traditionally, mustard is used for its stimulating, cleansing, and rejuvenating qualities. The warmth of the mustard assists in opening pores, helping the body to sweat out impurities. The powder can be blended with essential oils of wintergreen (antiseptic astringent), eucalyputus (antiseptic balsamic, cooling), rosemary (calming, soothing skin tonic) and thyme (antiseptic, stimulant). These natrual oils leave your skin feeling soothing and refreshed.

Indications: Fatigue, muscle and joint soresness, insomnia.

Equipment: Bathtub, shower, towels, mustard powder (ingredients: powdered mustard seed, essential oils of winter-green, eucalyptus, rosemary, thyme, sodium carbonate)

Procedure: Fill a tub two-thirds full with warm-hot water. Dissolve two large tablespoons of the powder into the bath. Assist client into bath, where he or she should soak for fifteen to twenty minutes. Assist client out of the bath and into a cool shower. Keep the shower brief. Allow client to rest, wrapped in a warm blanket.

Seaweed Powder Bath

Deep freezing and drying the seaweed (by lyophilisation) conserves the product's natural qualities in a way no other method can. It conserves mineral salts, vitamins, enzymes, and the aroma.

Effects: Stimulates blood circulation, helps eliminate toxins, aids in toning the skin, restores mineral salts and trace elements.

Equipment: Bathtub, shower, towels, seaweed powder.

Procedure: Prepare the bath by adding two ounces of seaweed powder to 40 to 50 gallons (150-200 litres) of warm water, 102°F. Assist client into bath, and ensure his or her comfort. Place a cool damp towel on client's forehead. Allow client to relax in the bath for fifteen to twenty minutes, or longer, if client is comfortable. Check on the client every ten minutes. Provide client with plenty of liquid to drink. A subsequent half-hour rest, with client wrapped in a warm bathrobe or blanket, will increase effectiveness of bath. The rest period prolongs perspiration and the consequent elimination of toxins. Follow with as cold a shower as possible.

Herbal Essential Oil Baths

Herbal bath oils are highly concentrated extracts that contain vitamins, hormones, antibiotics and antiseptics. In a warm bath the oils are absorbed through the skin, inducing deep relaxation that reduces stress, tension and muscle aches.

Equipment: Bathtub, towels, herbal essential oils.

Procedure: Prepare bath by adding two ounces of herbal oil to 40 to 50 gallons (150–200 litres) of warm water, 102°F. Assist client into bath and ensure his or her comfort. Place a cool, damp towel on client's forehead. Let client relax in tub for fifteen to twenty minutes or longer if client is comfortable. Check on the client every ten minutes. Provide client with plenty of liquid to drink.

Bicarbonated Bath

Bicarbonated minerals are effervescent salts. When added to warm bath water, they create an effervescent bath. They ease minor aches and pains and detoxify the skin.

Indications: Stress, minor pain, minor dermatological problems, high blood pressure, vegotonic and respiratory conditions, muscle fatigue.

Equipment: Bathtub, shower, towels, bicarbonate salts (ingredients: natrium hydrogen carbonate and aluminium sulphate).

Procedure: Fill bathtub two-thirds full with warm water, 86° to 98°F. Add bag one of bicarbonate–15 ounces (429 grams) of natrium hydrogen carbonate. Assist client into bath water. Add bag two of bicarbonate–18 ounces (508 grams) of aluminium sulphate pebbles. The bicarbonate development will begin. Let client bathe for twenty minutes, or until all pebbles are dissolved. Follow bath with a cool or cold shower. Let client rest, warmly wrapped, for thirty minutes.

Oxygen Bath

The oxygen-activated bath salts develop smooth pearl bubbles across the skin. They are very soothing and help release tension, increase physical vitality, regenerate the nervous and metabolic systems and improve blood circulation in arms and legs.

Equipment: Bathtub, shower, towels, oxygen salts (ingredients: natriumporcarbonate with 13.5 percent active oxygen).

Procedure: Dissolve the content of the salt, which is the oxygen carrier, in 97°F bath water. Assist client into the bath. Add the oxygen activator. Pearl-like oxygen bubbles will begin to form and cover the skin. Allow client to relax in bath for twenty minutes. Assist client out of bath and into a cool shower. Follow with rest, with client warmly wrapped, for one hour.

Underwater Pressure Massage

The therapeutic benefit of the underwater massage comes from the relaxing effect of warm water applied at variable force, particularly on deep-lying muscle layers, subcutaneous tissues, skin, and the abdominal organs (intestines).

In the underwater massage, the client lies relaxed in a large tub of warm water. A stream of water under pressure (ranging from 0.5 to a maximum of 7.0 bar absolute pressure units), is applied by means of a hose that has interchangeable nozzles.

Generally, the length of an underwater pressure massage is twenty to thirty minutes. It's necessary for the person to get used to the water for a few minutes before starting the massage. After the massage, the client may want a cold affusion to stimulate circulation. The client should then rest for approximately thirty minutes.

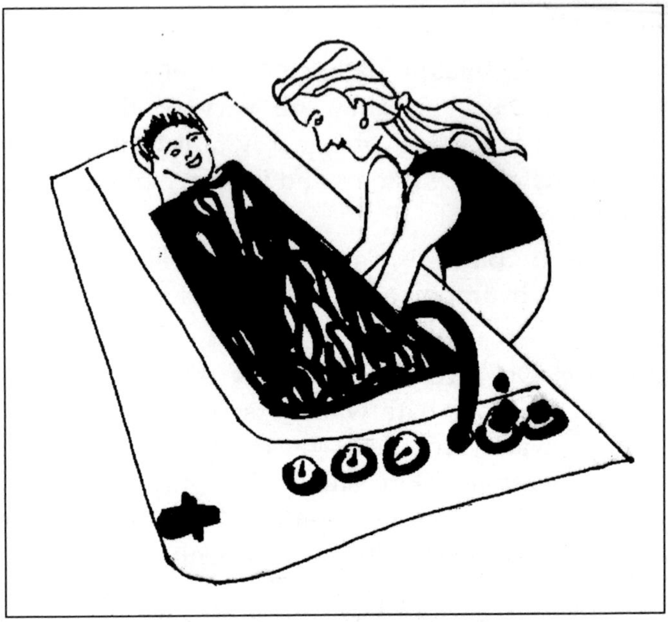

Underwater Pressure Massage

Sensitive areas of the body, such as the spinous processes of the spinal column bone spurs, genitalia, anus, back of the knees, and the female breasts should be avoided during the underwater massage. Similarly, the massage is not recommended for any recent athletic injuries; open wounds; hematomas in an acute state; effusions in the knee joints; acute muscle, ligament, and tendon pulls; and recent fractures.

Indications: Fractures, osteosynthesis, dislocation, sprains, contusions in the subacute stages after a client has been released, sciatica, lumbalgia, brachialgia, joint and scar contractures, myogeloses, degenerative spinal disorders, chronic joint rheumatism, muscular rheumatism, Bechterev's Disease (ankylosing spondylitis), scoliosis, flaccid and spastic paralyses.

The underwater massage can also be utilized for muscular hypertonia and for uninjured athletes as a warm-down massage after strenuous training and competition.

Contra-indications: Cardiovascular insufficiencies, venous disorders, thrombosis, varices.

Steam Vapour Bath

Heating water or a high temperature produces the gaseous state of water. Wet or dry (sauna) steam is invaluable in stimulating the skin and the resultant perspiration helps to evacuate stored toxins.

Equipment: Boiling kettle, electric home vaporizer or cold steam humidifier.

Indications: Sinus attacks, breathing problems, bronchitis, hoarseness, laryngitis.

Procedure: Prepare vaporizer. Add a few drops of compound or simple tincture of benzoin to the vaporizer lid.

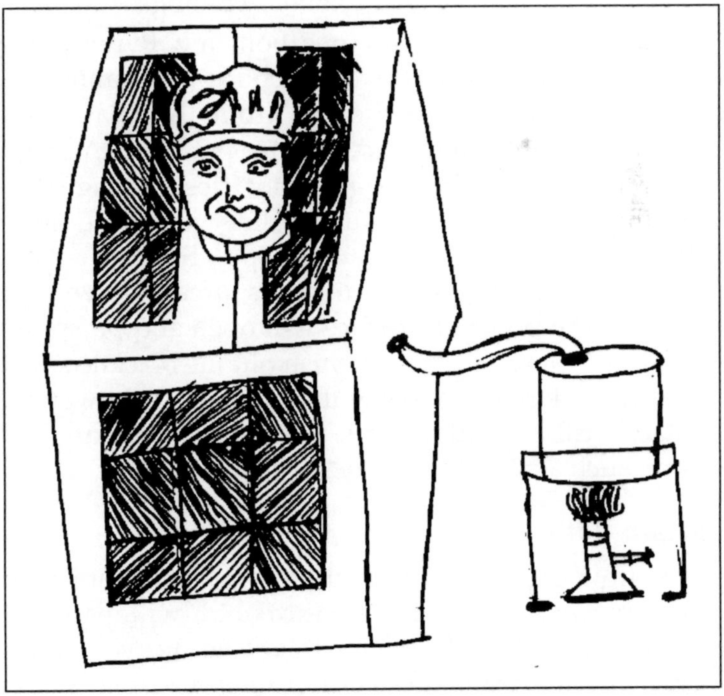

Steam Vapour Bath—Sauna Bath

(The tincture is made from a resin, so it will leave a gummy film, but it is very helpful in chest complaints and has the added advantage of being a cosmetic aid. It is also a remarkable aid in restoring the voice.) In the event there is no electric vaporizer available, boil water in a kettle, and keep it going by means of an electric tray, or some other safe arrangement. Create an improvised tent over the client's body and direct the steam so that the client does not get too wet or perspire. A large umbrella can be used. Occasionally sponge or use a cold mitten massage on, the client's body, as this will aid circulation and create a feeling of well-being.

Facials

To duplicate a professional facial, follow this procedure. This procedure is most useful for those with excessively oily skin. Do it in a non-drafty area to avoid chilling.

Procedure: Bring to a vigorous boil in a Pyrex pot two quarts of water to which two tablespoons of chamomile tea have been added. Remove the pot from the heat, place a newspaper on a table, and place the hot pot on the paper. Sit with your face above the pot (but not close enough to get burned). Improvise a tent by surrounding your head and the pot with a towel so that no steam escapes. Sit under the tent with eyes closed for five to ten minutes, breathing with your mouth open. The pores of the face will open and perspiration will pour out. Afterward, gently push out the blackheads with a cotton swab. Close the pores with a splash of cold water and sweep face with a cotton pad moistened with an herbal astringent, such as witch hazel.

Hot Steam Bath

A free flow of perspiration will often relieve the extreme pain of arthritis, gout, and sciatica and will ease other pain. Steam baths are often available in local gyms and are now available in steam rooms or pre-built sauna units for home.

Indications: Arthritis, fractures, sprains, sciatica, chronic low back pains, eliminates stored toxins.

Finnish Sauna

Many accident victims or arthritis clients find that the dry heat of the Finnish sauna helps them to function in a more normal manner. There is an intense but tolerable heat in the sauna room and this causes profuse perspiration within a few minutes. The ideal way to take a sauna is to perspire, then take a tepid of a cool shower, and then plunge into a cold pool of water. The total effect of these three water activities is a feeling of great cleanliness and exhilaration.

Indications: Fatigue, arthritis, after exercise, rheumatism, skin problems, poor circulation. The body soon develops a capacity to tolerate frequent saunas.

■

26

Baths of Different Organs

Organs like eyes, head, anus, vagina, spine ore given sepearate baths to cure specific problems. Here is a summary:

Eye Bath

It is necessary to take eye bath like other parts of the body. It cures eye diseases and increases eye-sight. There are two methods of taking eye bath.

First

Fill clean water in a bowl of glass or earth and keep it on a table or some high place. Dip your both eyes in this water. Keep on shutting and opening of your eyes in water upto 5 or 7 minutes, give them rest and avoid to go out in sunshine and avoid blows of wind. If something falls in eyes it comes out by

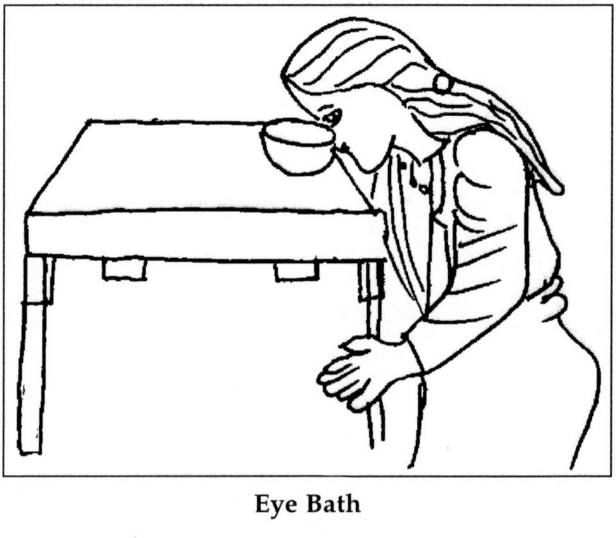

Eye Bath

eye bath. It relieves pain in eyes and calms down. Water for eye bath should be clean, cold and fresh. One should not take bath in the water of ponds, etc.

Second

Purchase an eye glass from the market. Fill it with clean water and open and shut your eyes in it by turn for five to seven minutes. Throw the water of eye glass after the bath of one eye. Fill it again for the bath of the other eye. Rose water, Trifla water and solution of Fitkari are also used.

Head Bath

Take this bath weekly or after ten days. Wash your head with cold water, rubbing the scalp with your fingers for five to seven minutes. This bath gives relief in all diseases concerned with head as headache, falling of hair, untimely greying of hair, deafness, madness and weakness of the eyes. To remove dryness of hair, one should massage head with pure mustard oil twice a week.

Anus Bath

The patient takes cold water in a vessel. He takes out a little water in his hand and throws it at the exact place from where he passes stool. Then he rubs that place with his hand vigorously. He repeats it from two to five minutes. After that he pours his finger in cold water and inserts it in anus and takes out. He performs this action for a minute.

This therapy clears the bowl and removes constipation. Persons, who do not like to take enema, can take the benefits of enema through this anus bath.

Vaginal Bath

Vaginal tube is availabe in market just like an anema instrument. Water from an enema instrument through this vagina tube is inserted in vagina and vagina is cleaned and washed by this water. It strengthens the vagina and ovary too. All diseases concerned with vagina are cured by it.

Madu Basti—Bath of Penis

Like vagina bath tip of penis is washed by stream of cold water. It removes the diseases of male organ and urinary diseases of bladder.

Bath of Spine

There are many methods of spinal bath. Some of them are as following:

First

Wet a large towel with cold water and rinse it. Catch both the ends of the towel with both hands and take them to the back side. Now rub the backbone with towel. Wet the towel afer one or two minutes. Do it for five minutes and wash head with cold water. Finish it by cold rubbing.

Second

Make a cushion one foot wide, two feet long and half inch in thickness of a dhoti or clothsheet. Spread it on clean floor or a wooden bed and wet this cushion with cold water well. Lie on it with naked back. The cushion should be under back and the head and feet should be away from it. Now cover the whole body with a blanket except head. Lie down under the blanket until warm. At last, wash the head with cold water and finish this bath by cold rubbing bath.

Third

Keep feet on a board and sit naked with folded legs. Ask someone to pour cold water with a jug in a thin stream continuously for five minutes on your backbone. After that, rub that place with a dry cloth. Wash the head with cold water and take cold rubbing bath.

Fourth

Take a tub six feet in length, three feet in breadth and six inches in height. Fill it upto three inches with cold water. Lie down on back naked in it and cover the tub and body with blanket. Keep your feet out of the tub. Wrap a wet cloth on chest and abdomen. After eyery two minutes sit in the tub and dry your back with a dry towel and lie down in the tub again. Continue it for 10 minutes, wash your head with cold water and do cold rubbing bath.

Friction Hip Bath

It is called Cune bath also as it is named in the name of its inventor Lui Cune, a resident of town Lipzig of Germany. It is necessary to rub the lower part of abdomen in this bath, so it is called friction bath.

Method: Take a chair type tub. Fill it with water. The water should reach thighs and navel on sitting. The temperature of water should be 64 to 68°F. It may be fresh water of a well which is generally of this temperature. One should not use freezing cold water for this bath. It is called cold back bath also.

Sit in the tub naked suddenly. Keep your back on chair. By doing this, spine is also bathed. This doubles the process of disease prevention. Keep your feet outside of the tub on a stool, brick or ckowki. Cover every part of the body with a cloth outside water except head and face. Generally, for natural treatment, it is necessary first to take bath in lukewarm water having temperature 100°F and afterwards in cold water. It is sufficient to cover the dry parts of the body with a large

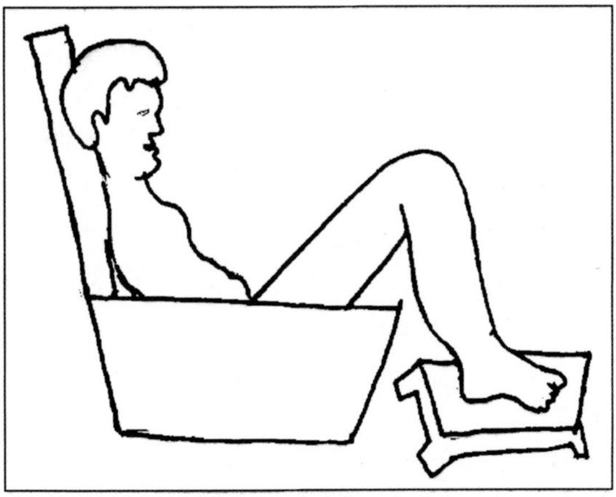

Kati Snan—Anus Bath

blanket (if the patient is suffering from fever, he can bathe without blanket). If the feet remain cold, wear socks.

It is good to make the lower part of abdomen under navel, warm by dry rubbing before sitting in the tub. One should start it without wearing clothes.

After sitting in the tub, take a small khadi towel or a folded piece of soft jute in your right hand and wet it. Rub it from right to left and left to right on navel in half circular way. Simultaneously both the hips upto anus and thighs upto outer part of pelvis organ should be rubbed with it. This rubbing or friction should be a bit forcefully but avoiding brushing of the skin. Lower part of abdomen is proper for this friction bath, as our intestines are situated in this part of abdomen in which whole excreta is stored. To cure and clean intestines and kidney by making their work of excretion easy and proper, this friction bath is best remedy. In beginning this bath should continue upto 5 to 10 minutes. Increase the duration by two minutes after each two or three days. The duration of this friction should not be more than twenty minutes.

Old diseases can be aggravated by this bath and it is a good symptom. After bath one should come out of the tub and wash the body upto back with cold water. Wash both arms, head and at last both the feet. After friction bath one should take full bath and rub the body with a dry towel. Wear clothes and try to warm the body by doing exercise in open air, walking or dry massaging. The body can be warmed by wearing woollen clothes or by covering the body by a blanket.

Special precautions

- The lady whose menses have commenced, should not take this bath upto four days.
- It is beneficial to take friction bath punctually at a fixed time.
- Old persons can take this bath in lukewarm water.
- One should observe chastity during the period of this bath.

- It benefits more if the bandage of clay or earth is laid on the abdomen prior to it.
- It is not beneficial to take this bath if you are on fast.
- One should take this friction bath regularly on a punctual time for a month and then it should be stopped for a week. Again start it and continue it in this manner until the disease is fully cured.
- In serious diseases this bath should be taken at early intervals many times and in old diseases once or twice only. It should continue until the disease is fully cured.

Benefits

1. It removes constipation certainly.
2. It improves blood circulation in liver, spleen and intestines which help in keeping the diseases away.
3. This friction hip bath improves the whole nervous system which helps in curing all diseases of body.
4. The patient suffering from piles should use tapid water to sit in.

Friction Mahen Snan (Cune)

This bath is called sex organ's bath. This is beneficial in female diseases also.

Method for Females

A stool of one foot height is kept in the bath tub. Cold water is filled upto the level of stool. The body should sit naked on the stool and keep the feet on same bench or stool outside the tub. She should take a small towel or thick handkerchief. She should wash again and again softly and continuously the outer portion of the child-procreating organ. She should not touch inner side of the organ. The skin of that place should not be rubbed vigorously. It should be rubbed from five to twenty minutes. Rub the body from neck to hips slowly with a wet cloth. Above portion of body and feet should keep dry. If the hips get wet, it does not affect the effect of bath. The dry portion of the body should be warmed by exercise or by covering the body with some quilt after the bath.

One should not take this bath in menstruation. Water should be cold but not freezing cold.

Method for Males

Male should sit on the stool kept in the bath tub filled with water naked just like a female. He should catch the tip of penis by two fingers of left hand and wash it with the wet cloth again and again gently and slowly.

Persons whose skin of the tip of penis has been cut off due to Khatna (a ceremony among Mohammedans) or due to some other reason should wash the skin between testicles. Keep the lower part of the back under water upto three inches. It would wet the hips. But the legs and above portion of the body should be dry. One should try to avoid wetting the major portion of the testicles.

After taking Mahen Snan (Cune bath) once or twice, generally the symptoms of the disease at the spot of friction or nearby may appear. It is a good sign. If some portion of the hips remains drowned in water, it shows the effect of bath soon. After bath the patient should walk in open ground for twenty minutes to warm himself. One can be warmed by covering his body with a blanket or quilt.

Benefits: For this Mahen bath the procreating organ was selected, because many nerves end at the tips of this organ. It is very scientific to give the bath to this part of the body. It affects the nerves of each and every corner of the body.

This bath removes the heat of impure substance in body. It strengthens nervous system and thus paves the way for healthy life. It pacifies mind and is very beneficial if it is taken before sleep.

Other things of this bath are like friction hip bath.

■

27

Aromatic Bath

Bathing no doubt, is not merely a ritual but it has multiple benefits also, as water has remedial and relaxing properties. When bathing is preceded by an essential oil massage, it has multifold salutary effects. In Hindu religion, bathing is a way to healthy and hygienic life. Even in Greek and Roman cultures bathing was accorded a significantly important place. Bathing with essential oils can calm the agitated nerves, stimulate blood circulation, relax and deodorise the foul smelling body, uplift mood and remove the harmful foreign matters that cling to the body. There is a large list of essential oils out of which you can choose the most suitable oil(s) depending on your individual requirement and state of health.

Needless to remind that aromatic baths can help a lot in mitigating or even removing , the conditions like stiffness of joints, pains and aches, fatigue, colds, headache, tone and condition the skin, relieve tension and anxiety and detoxify the body, remove foul odour and perspiration etc.

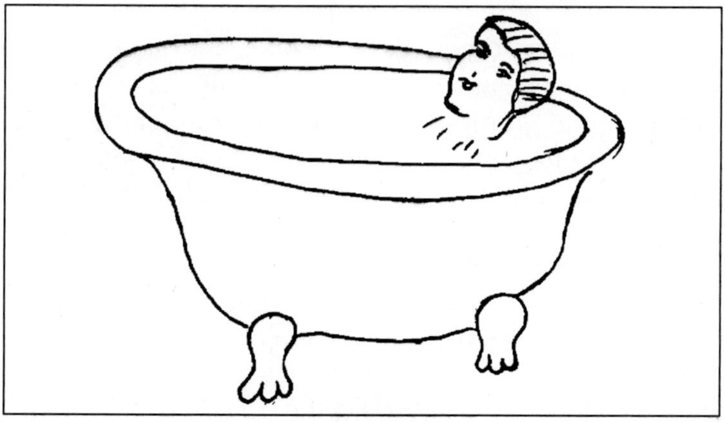

Aromatic Bath

Essential Oils for Specific Problems of Health

Oils for Relaxation

Basil, Bergamot, Cedarwood, Chamomile, Frankincense, Hyssop, Juniper, Lavender, Marjoram, Melissa, Neroli, Patchouli, Rose, Sage, Sandalwood, Ylang-Ylang.

Oils for Stimulation

Cypress, Eucalyptus, Fennel, Geranium, Juniper, Lavender, Lemon, Lemon grass, Peppermint, Pine, Rosemary, Thyme.

Oils for Rheumatism/Arthritis

Chamomile, Eucalyptus, Juniper, Lavender, Rosemary, Thyme.

Oils for Eczema

Chamomile, Geranium, Hyssop, Juniper, Myrrh, Rosemary.

Oils for Dermatitis

Chamomile, Hyssop, Lavender.

Oils for Psoriasis

Bergamot, Chamomile, Lavender.

If you study the above list, you can easily make out that oils like Chamomile, Juniper, Rosemary, Lavender have been repeated quite often which implies that related disorders can be treated by using a specific oil for various applications and uses.

Use of Oils for the Bath

Essential oils make a bath both aromaticaly and therapeuticaly. They sink into the skin quickly and thoroughly apart from giving floral and herbal fragrances. If oil is added directly to the bath, it will float on the surface of bathing water, thus imparting the full aromatic benefits to you. To yield better and quicker results you can mix oil(s) in a base oil (like apricot kernel, sweet almond oil, Evening Primrose or Jujoba base oils) and then, disperse the blended oil through the water.

While choosing oils make sure that they do not counter balance one another, rather they should complement and enhance the effect of other oils. Do not blend more than three essential oils at a time. Mix 5 drops of each type of oil to a 15 ml. of skin-softening oil.

Temperature of a Running Bath

Time and temperature are important in a bath. Highly hot water is harmful and damaging in some diseases even though it increases heart beat and allows the capillaries and blood vessels to expand. Pregnant ladies, persons having high blood pressure, dandruff, piles, vericose veins must avoid hot water due to the above given reasons. Spend around 15-20 minutes in bath. Add dilute oils to water when the bath tub/buckets is full, and never earlier, as these oils evaporate quickly.

Relaxation Bath

Mark Evans suggests – "To calm yourself after a fraughtful day or to prepare yourself for a peaceful night's sleep, turn your bathroom into a private sanctury. Keep the light soft, if possible, or use an eye-mask or burn aromatic candles. Support your head with a bath pillow, close your eyes and inhale deeply. Concentrate on your breathing, empty your mind and let the oil soothe away your stresses and strains. After a 15-20 minute soak, get out slowly and wrap yourself in a large warm towel."

Stimulating Bath

In this context Mark Evans adds—"Stimulating Bath is the best for the morning to get you started or to revive you before an evening out. Keep the water fairly cool and use an invigorating bath to rub down.

The Weekly Scalp Massage

For dry and sensitive skin: Massage 1 tsp warm sesame oil into scalp for 10 minutes. Wrap head in hot towel and leave on for five to ten minutes. Do once a week for sensitive skin and twice a week for dry skin or dandruff. The best time for this treatment is first thing in the morning or before bed. Massage increases circulation to the scalp. Therefore, do not do this massage right after a meal, when the blood supply is needed for proper digestion.

For oily skin: With head down, dry brush hair 50 times from roots to end to spread natural oils.

Body Baths for Glow

In many cultures throughout history, the bath has been-and is-an important ritual for purification of body and mind. In the Vedic tradition, we honour the temple statues with a "five nectar" bath of milk, honey, ghee, yoghurt and banana, which are the five perfect foods according to Ayurveda.

Baths are holy-that is, they purify us and make us whole. Indeed, there is nothing so rejuvenating to the spirit and relaxing to the body than a leisurely soak in the tub. Consequently, Ayurveda considers the bath to be a vital part of daily life. Of course, the pace of modern life leaves most people with barely enough time to take a quick shower once a day. Nevertheless, taking half an hour to yourself once a week for a cleansing and nourishing body bath is really the least you can do for your health and peace of mind. It is also one of the fastest and easiest ways to increase your glow.

■

28

Showers and Steam Showers

Showers include all applications of water or steam that are administered under pressure. Showers are divided into cold, neutral, warm and hot. Hot showers and extended showers are preferred for rheumatic disorders. Showers can be rain or fan, with a gentle low pressure, and used in various temperatures.

For the athlete, warm showers after training or competition have a generally lossseing and relaxing effect, in addition to being cleansing. Cold showers have a tonic effect on the blood vessels and are a good way to conclude warm showers. Steam showers can be used to improve muscular recovery after competition. The steam shower is also suited for the treatment of residual damage, such as occurs in contractures, scars and rheumatic disorders.

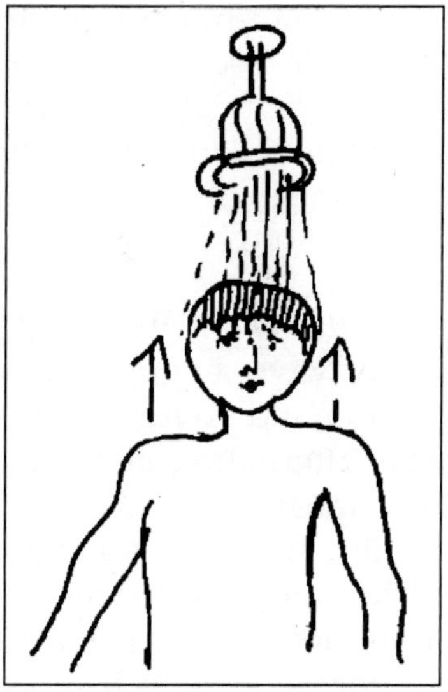

Shower Bath

In a steam shower, the steam is sprayed onto the skin at a mild comfortable pressure and a temperature of about 110°F. The treating person should keep a distance of six feet from the client, as the steam can otherwise scald.

Cold Shower

The shower is used as cold as, and as long as, the client can tolerate it. The endurance to cold will increase as the procedure is prolonged.

Contra-indications: Cardiovascular instability.

Effects: Overcomes fatigue, tonic effect, reduces elevated body temperature.

Hot Shower

A light spray-rain shower for two to five minutes with temperature from 100°F to 104°F eases neuralgic pain and comforts the body.

Contraindications: Any form of swelling, lymph edema.

Effects: Prepares client for a cold treatment, alleviates pain, soothes irritated skin.

Neutral Shower

A light gentle-spray shower for four to six minutes in lukewarm (92–97°F), body-temperature water relaxes the body by contracting the circulatory blood system. The reaction is similar to that with a long neutral bath.

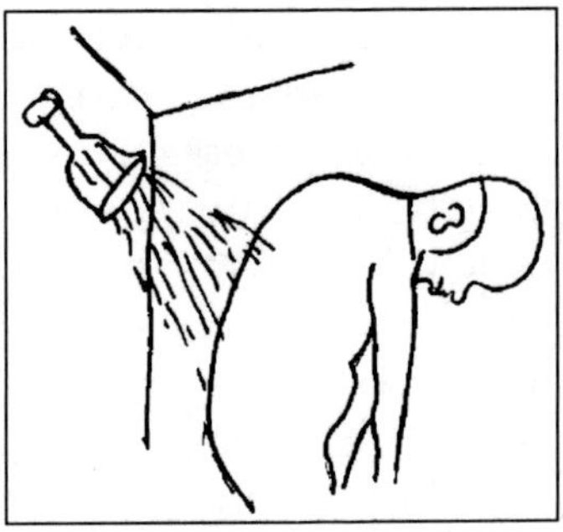

Alternate Hot and Cold Shower

Always begin with the hot shower and do not shock the body. The alternating temperature has the most body hardening and conditioning effect. Equal amounts of hot and cold water or unequal amounts can be applied with emphasis on the water.

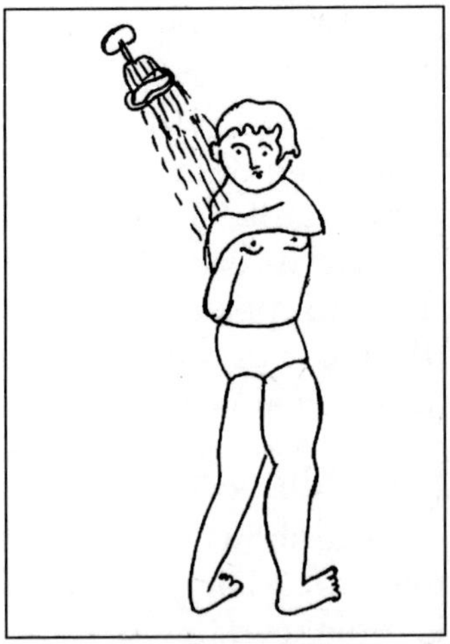

Shower Bath

Swiss Shower

This cascading vertical body spray shower has nine or more sprays. It creates a gentle or vigorous rain shower from the ankles to the shoulders from above.

It is commonly used before and/or after a herbal body wrap, skin exfoliation and massage therapy. The treatment provides relief from symptoms oftension, insomnia and stress. A true shower treatment is actually a full body alternating-temperature hydro-massage performed by the effect of the shower heads.

Indicaions: Chronic back pain, insomnia, vascular instability.

Contra-indications: Cardiovascular insufficiencies, venous disorders, thrombosis, varices.

Temperature: 103°F to 70°F, to 103°F to 65°F, and so on.

Vichy Shower

The Vichy shower therapy was originally created for clients with apoplexy, paraplegia, quadriplegia and cardiovascular insufficiencies. The Vichy shower is a horizontal shower bar with shower nozzles arranged so that the entire body, situated on a table, is covered with a gentle water stream. The Vichy shower therapy is a form of hydromassage with a temperature of about 105°F or contrast temperature (warm-cool) application. For optimal vascular results, the client is brushed with a soft bristle brush.

Indications: Chronic fatigue, mild hypertension, lymphatic congestion, skin exfoliation and cleansing.

Contra-indications: Vascular instability, open skin ailments, lymph edema, pregnancy.

Washing Down With a Wet Cloth or Mitten

Ablution, performed with a wet cloth, is the midlest form of kneipp water application. Ablution differs from usual cleansing procedures. The washing procedure is divided into whole and partial body washings. Treatment should take place in a draft-free, warm room. A coarse linen wash cloth is recommended for the procedure. Water should be applied evenly to the body parts being washed. The stimulating effect of the washing (especially on the skin's circulation) may water. Use one part vinegar to two parts water.

Effects: Enhances blood circulation, relaxes, activates the production of heat in the body. The toxic substances in the blood will be increasingly eliminated and even prevented in the limbs.

Washing of Upper Extremities, Chest, and Back

Indications: Stress syndrome, dysfunctional thermoregulatory system, rheumatism, colds, fever.

Contra-indications: Oversensitivity to cold.

Effect: Thoughens the skin, improves circulation, stimulates metabolism.

Equipment: Coarse linen washcloth.

Procedure: Dip a coarse linen washcloth in cold water. Wash the right arm-first the exterior, from the shoulder to the hand, then the interior to the armpit. Move to left arm-same procedure. Stroke across the chest and then clockwise across the abdomen. The back side is rubbed down with severel strokes. Ablution should be performed as quickly as possible. Do not dry. Have client dressed in pajamas and assist him or her into a warm bed.

Water additives: Vinegar.

Washing of Lower Extremities, Buttocks

Indications: Stress syndrome, dysfunction of body's thermoregulatory system (rhemuatism, cold, fever), poor circulation, insomnia, varicose veins, thryoid overactivity.

Contra-indications: Oversensitivity to cold, bladder or kidney infection, inflammation or infection of the female pelvic organs.

Effects: Toughens skin, reduces insomnia, stimulates metabolism, promotes digestive process.

Equipment: Coarse linen washcloth, cold water.

Procedure: Dip a coarse linen washcloth into cold water. Wash the right leg – first exterior front. Move to the left leg front. Then wash the right leg back. Move to the left leg back. End with the soles of the feet. Ablution should be performed as quickly as possible. Do not dry. Have client dressed in either a nightdress or pajamas and get into a warm bed.

Water additives: Vinegar.

Washing Down of Arms and Legs

Indications: Fever, acute infections.

Contra-indications: Oversensitivity to cold, cold hands or feet.

Effects: Reduces fever, increases perspiration, improves circulation, refreshes.

Equipment: Coarse linen washcloth, cold water.

Procedure: Assist client into bed, then dip a coarse washcloth into cold water. Washing down begins with lower part of the legs or lower part of the arms. Ablution should be performed as quickly as possible. Do not dry. Cover client well with a blanket. If the client feels warm again, repeat the procedure. The procedure can be repeated several times in an hour.

Water Additives: Vinegar.

Body Wraps

Every wrap has it's own specific effect on the system. However, all wraps relax muscles, break up and absorb body toxins, and stimulate the whole organism. The major function of the wrap is to stimulate the skin, which in turn influences the body temperature, the nervous system, blood circulation, and the immune system. The effect of the wrap depends on its duration.

Types of Wrap: Chest wrap, throat wrap, lumbar wrap, shawl wrap, foot wrap, short wrap, calf wrap, leg wrap, hand wrap, wet socks.

Wrap Material: Coarse linen cloth (interior cloth) lies on the skin, moist. Cotton cloth (middle cloth) dry on the edges, two centimeters wider than the interior cloth. Wool blanket (exterior cloth) dry on the edges, one centimeter smaller than the middle cloth.

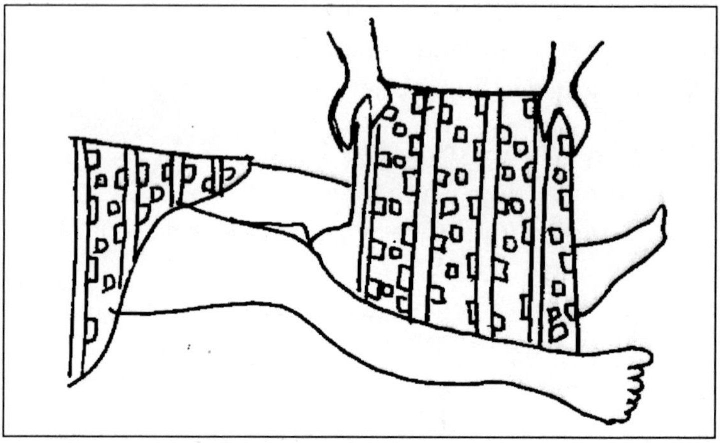

Calf Wrap

Rules about Body Wraps

1. They can be administered cold, tepid, or hot.
2. Additives such as vinegar, argillaceous earth (clay), salt and dried herbs are effective.
3. Digestive tract should be cleared prior to wrap.
4. Hot wraps must be applied as hot as possible, while avoiding burns.
5. The wrap must be removed as quickly as possible.
6. After the wrap, the client should rest for thirty to sixty minutes.
7. The client should not read or watch television.
8. All wraps must fit snugly around the body.
9. Each cloth is wrapped in the same manner.

■

29

Magnetised Water and Oil

When the properties of a magnet are absorbed in water by continuous contact between the two, the water gets magnetised and gives relief in innumerable diseases when taken internally for some considerable time.

Magnetised water can be easily prepared at home.

Ingredients

1. Two round shaped powerful magnets. (Magnets should be of 2 to 3 thousand gauss).
2. Fresh drinking water.
3. Two glasses.
4. A big and clean glass bottle.

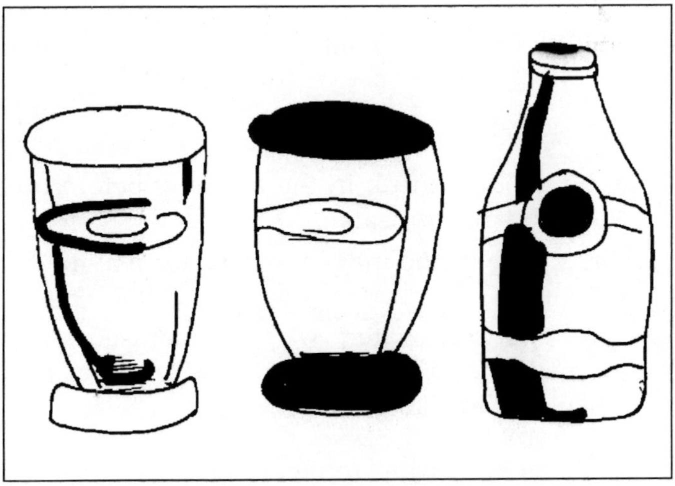

Magnetised Water

Method

Boil one litre of fresh water and cool it. Fill both the glasses with this water. Keep the North pole magnet towards the North and the South pole magnet towards the south direction on the wooden plank. Keep the glasses on the centre of the magnets. Cover the glasses with plastic or wooden lids and let them remain on the magnets for 24 hours. Magnet waves pass through glass and have their effect on the water. Thus, the water gets magnetised. Then the water of both the glasses is transferred to a clean glass bottle.

The magnets should not be kept in water. The bottle should be filled with magnetised water upto neck. Stir it well before use.

Dosage

1. For one year old infant	One spoon
2. For a baby of two years	Two spoons
3. For a child of 3 years	Three spoons at a time, thrice daily
4. For a child of 12 years	Half cup of water
5. For adult and old person	Two ounces (50 ml.) at a time, twice daily

Time

It may be good to drink in the morning before breakfast and after both the major meals.

In fever, a dose of the magnetised water may be taken at every two hours.

Note—Magnetised water, with magnetised properties becomes a medicine and should not be taken in excessive quantities like simple plain water.

Beneficial Effects of Magnetised Water

Scientists have proved that the magnetised water, prepared from the healing vibrations of permanent magnets, helps in almost all diseases and is especially beneficial in the disorders of the digestive, nervous and urinary system. Main benefits of it are as follows:

1. Magnetised water improves digestion, increases appetite and reduces excess of acids and bile.
2. If improves movements of bowels and expels poison, unwanted salts and morbidity from the body.
3. The magnetised water helps in kidney troubles. If urine is stopped, administration of 25 ml. (one ounce) of the magnetised water mixed with equal quantity of plain water in quite succession of 5 to 10 minutes for 8 to 10 times will make the patient pass urine.
4. It helps in washing out the salts and stones from kidneys and gall-bladder.
5. The magnetised water is effective in treatment of all sorts of fever, all kinds of pains, asthma, bronchitis, colds, coughs, headaches, etc.
6. The magnetised water helps in clearing the clogged arteries. It normalises circulatory system and helps in regulating the functioning of the heart.
7. Magnetised water is administered to women to regulate their cycle of menses.

Magnetised Oil

Oil can be magnetised and made more powerful with healing characteristics like water. Yellow mustard oil, sesame oil or groundnut oil can be magnetised.

Oil magnetised by North pole assists in curing paralysis, baldness, weakness etc. Oil magnetised by South pole gives relief in skin diseases, diseases of the ear, all sorts of pains, insomnia etc.

Oil magnetised by both the poles is effective for massage of the hair and the body. Head and the soles of the feet should be massaged by the magnetised oil.

Keep the oil magnetised by North pole in a bottle of red colour in sunshine for eight hours. Similarly keep the oil magnetised by South pole in a bottle of blue colour in sunshine for eight hours. The bottles should be tightly corked. Thus the oil becomes more potent.

■

30

Water in Early Morning

Water is panacea for chronic and incurable diseases. Rise early from bed. Do not wash your face and mouth as you do normally. Sit comfortably and drink four large glasses of water. Do not take any thing for 45 minutes. You can wash your face and brush your mouth after drinking water.

Always drink water after an hour of breakfast and meals. Regular intake of water in early morning gives relief in following diseases:

1. Diabetes
2. Acne, Boils
3. Headache
4. Blood pressure
5. Old age and wrinkles
6. Arthritis
7. Paralysis problem of ladies
8. Anaemia
9. Heart diseases, Faintness
10. Cold, Cough, Asthma, Bronchitis
11. Obesity
12. Meningitis
13. Disorders of liver
14. Tuberculosis
15. Disorders of the eye
16. Irregular menstruation
17. Urinary problems, Stones, etc.
18. Hyperacidity, Asthma, Bronchitis
19. Gastric trouble and diseases concerned with back, Spine
20. Cancer of ovary
21. Swelling, Fever
22. Digestive disorders
23. Piles
24. Diseases caused by Vata, Pitta, Cough.
25. Mental weakness, etc.

If sick persons or soft natured persons with a delicate physique are unable to take four glasses of water at a stretch, they should start from one or two glasses and then gradually they should start taking four glasses. Take four glasses of water regularly. Experiments have proved that different diseases can be cured within the time given below by its regular use:

Hypertension	–	Within one month
Gastric trouble	–	Within ten days
Cancer	–	Within six months
Constipation	–	Within ten days
Diabetes	–	Within one month
TB	–	Within three months
Leucorrhoea	–	Within one month
Paralysis	–	Within three months

Other diseases described above may be cured within four to six months according to their nature. Drinking four glasses of water does not have any ill-effects on health. Only urge to pass urine will be great and you will pass urine in large quantities frequently. Passing of stool will be easy and complete. It will facilitate the expulsion of the accumulated waste matter very effectively and leave you fresh. Besides hydrotherapy certain other measures or house hold remedies are also advised for such disorders.

Some Important Facts

1. Never drink water before passing urine or just after passing urine.
2. Passing urine after meals prevents formation of stones.
3. Stand on forefoot and then pass urine. This posture prevents formation of stones.
4. Water contained in copper vessel is hundred times more useful.
5. Take juice of one lemon in a glass of warm water before going to bed. It gives relief in Coryza.

6. Take juice of one lemon and tea spoon of honey in warm water in morning. It helps in curing obesity and improves complexion.
7. In early morning, chew five leaves of Neem (Azadiracta indica) and Holy Tulsi (Ocimum basilum) and drink a glass of water after chewing these leaves. This can prevent you from carcinoma (Cancer) too.
8. Take a little rice (raw—one or two tea spoons) with a glass of water to cure liver disorders.
9. The water kept in a Shankh for a whole night is remedy for Stammering speech. Continue this for four to six months.

Role of Water on Stomach

There is secretion of stomachic juice in stomach to digest food. The more genuine the stomachic juice, the better digestion of food.

If someone takes liquid whether it is water, wine or beer, the stomachic juice will not remain genuine. It would be adulterated by the intake of water, wine or beer and would not be effective in digestion of food.

Similarly, if some person takes water six or eight times while taking his meal, it would liquidate stomachic juice so much that it would not be able to act as digestive juice.

Do not take water at all during meals. If you have to take it, take very small quantity of it, so that genuine stomachic juice may be absorbed in all eaten food.

If you feel thirsty after one hour or more of taking food, please take water in limited quantity. Body especially stomach needs water at interval from time to time to liquidate its juice, to increase its quantity and to absorb the solid material (food). The body itself informs whenever it needs it. Sometimes, the desire to take water is slow and sometimes it is very fast. One should be particular about intake whether it is from healthy or sick stomach. One should take it as much as it is sufficient and good for health.

It should be taken at equal intervals of time especially when one is suffering from fever. One should not take a glass of water at a stretch but each five or ten minutes in less quantity. Intake of water at a stretch by a patient of fever, will not quench his thirst, rather it would increase other symptoms of illness.

Water taken in less quantity is at once accepted and absorbed by stomach. Repetition of its intake at each half-an-hour produces juice in more quantity and removes whole dullness and constipation by flowing in body and intestines. It cools them also.

One can use luke-warm water or cold water according to its taste.

Use of Water

1. Saline water is necessary in dehydration caused by cholera, fever, diabetes, diarrhoea, etc.
2. It is useful to take water with salt, sugar, lemon and honey. Patients of kidney diseases should use water with salt in supervision of some naturopath.
3. Some of vegetables, water of pulse, sharbat of lemon and juice etc. contain water. They give us minerals and salts along with water.

■

31

Fango and Mustard Pack

Mustard powder, when made into a paste with a touch of water and flour and applied in a cloth on to lightly oiled skin, has unique power of bringing blood to the surface of the skin. It quickly heats up the area, and, as the blood rushes to the skin surface, even the worst congestion diminishes.

Indications: Internal congestion, lumbago, neuritis, poor local circulation, bronchitis, sciatica.

Procedure: Prepare a large linen or cotton cloth by folding the cloth in thirds. In a bowl, mix one cup of dry, powdered mustard with tepid water until it has creamy consistency. Increase the amount of power according to the amount of poultice needed. Place the mustard paste on a paper towel. Fold the towel and make a pack, and place it in the folded linen or cotton cloth. Heat the pack by placing a hot water bottle on it. If the client has sensitive skin, oil the skin lightly with olive or vegetable oil. Place a thin cloth on the area, and apply the mustard pack. Cover the area with a blanket. At first the heat may seem intense, but then it lessens. As the skin became very red, the pack can be transferred from area, of the chest to the upper back (in case of bronchitis) or to other areas of intense pain.

Duration: Apply the pack to each area for ten minutes. The entire teatment should last half-hour.

Hot and Cold Fango (Mud) and Clay Packs

Hot sand, hot fango packs and clay packs have been used for centuries by different cultures to relieve joint pain. The material used is either organic volcanic ash, peal from bags, mineral sea mud or clay from high mineral areas. All of these substances are availabe in powder form. Fango (mud) packs have extracting ability because the mineral content increases the heat and chemical action on the skin. Because clay and/or earth draw out poisons, such packs not only soften the skin and release tension around joints, but also absorb internal toxic or pathogenic material.

Indications: Chronic rheumatism, chronic neuralgia, chronic pain, non-acute arthritis, muscle spasms, chronic sciatica.

Contra-indications: Small application of clay or mud will vitalize the entire body, but immersion mineral mud baths are contraindicated in cases of heart disease, diabetes, high blood pressure or arteriosclerosis.

Procedure: Heat up the mud powder. Add water to soften it. Spread this in a one- or two-inch thickness on a soft cotton cloth, slightly larger than the area you wish to cover. Place the hot mud directly on the hurt area. Cover the area with a dry light weight cloth. Leave on until it dries (fifteen to thirty minutes). Rinse off with warm water, then splash with a little cool water. Remove the dried mud by sponging or showering it off. Follow with a rain or needle shower. Dry gently with a mild cloth. If the body is still heated, keep the area warm and dry afterward.

Fango Moor Pack (German)

Ingredients: Natural Moor-Peloid from the moorfields of northern Germany

Indications for Hot Pack

Application: Subacute and chronic conditions of rheumatism, degenerative joint and spinal conditions, soft tissue rheumatism, postacute traumas of joints and muscles, lack of functional blood circulation, chronic pain, discomfort in the abdominal region.

Contra-indications for Hot Pack

Application: Acute inflammation, trauma, bleeding, edema, insufficiencies in vascular capillaries and vessels, elevated body temperature, fever, sensitive skin areas, acute skin conditions, skin burns.

Indications for Cold Pack

Application: Acute conditions of rheumatism, degenerative joint and spinal conditions, soft tissue rheumatism, acute traumas of joints and muscles, acute inflammation of organs in the abdominal region, augmentive therapy in venous and lymphatic vascular symptoms, fever.

Contra-indications for Cold Pack

Application: Insufficiencies in vascular capillaries and vessels, local and general skin sensitivity to cold.

Procedure: Apply pack to the skin. Hot pack application temperature is 107°F or more, according to tolerance. Cold pack application temperature is 60°F or less, according to tolerance. Apply pack for twenty to thirty minutes. Client should rest after application for twenty to thirty minutes.

Parafango (Paraffin Fango) Pack

Investigations aimed at improving the thermophysical conditions of fango, which would make the application easier and raise the basic hygienic conditions when thermal fango packs were applied, led to the development of Parafango by Professor Hesse in Hambrug, Germany. Introduced as a treatment in 1952, the preparation has since become widely known in practice and literature in Europe. Parafango is compounded of dried fango and paraffins with different fusing points. It also contains minute additions of talcum and magnesium oxide in order to prevent the fango from precipitating in the melted paraffins, as well as to heighten the plasticity and the malleablitiy of the material. Parafango melts at (140°F–158°F) to an easy-to-spread paste that, exactly within the range of its temperature of application, constitutes an extremely plastic mass that is easily molded to any part of the body at 122°F. The application of hot Parafango packs on parts of the body's surface is a purely thermal process.

Indications: Inflammatory rheumatism (declining acute rheumatism and rheumatoid arthritis, anchylosing spondylitis), degenerative rheumatism (osteo arthritis, intervertebral discopathies, non-articular rheumatism such as fibrositis myalgia, painful shoulder), dermatology (psoriatic arthropaty, scleroderma).

Contra-indications: Acute neuritis, acute primary rheumatoid arthritis, recent thrombophlebitis and eczema, all forms of heart and circulation deficiencies, high grade hypertension, angina pectoris, distinct vegetative dystonia, and convalescence.

Procedure: Local packings: On one or two larger joints, a small area of torso.

Part packs: On three or four large joints, entire extremities, back and abdomen or pelvic packs.

Large packs: Entire extremities, back with abdominal pack.

Alpine Flower Haypack

Indications: Area with muscular tension and/or joint discomfort, degeneration of the joints, degeneration of the spine or acute bronchitis

Contra-indications: Heart disease, inflamed treatment area.

Effects: Relaxes, increass blood circulation, reduces pain, calms.

Equipment: 1 wool blanket, 1 linen cloth, 1 meadow flower herbal pack.

Procedure: Moisten the herbal pack with water. Place herbal pack in a steamer or in a hydroinfuser. Steam the pack for approximately thirty minutes. Remove the haypack carefully from the steamer and shake it with both hands. Apply the haypack carefully. Observe the skin's reaction to the pack. Gradually wrap tighter. After wrapping, cover client with a blanket. Remove the pack before it cools down (usually forty-five minutes). Have client rest for thirty to sixty minutes after the treatment. Neck Haypack—Hot Temperature.

Indications: Tightness in the neck, cervical syndrome.

Contra-indications: Neuritis, inflammation of the skin in the treatment area.

Effects: Relaxes muscles, reduces spasms, increases blood circulation, stimulates metabolism, reduces pain.

Equipment: 1 wool blanket, 1 linen cloth, 1 meadow flower haypack.

Procedure: Apply the hot haypack tightly onto the neck. Be careful not to burn the skin. In order to prevent heat from escaping, wrap the haypack snugly. Leave on as long as the pack feels warm.

Lumber Haypack—Hot Temperature

Indications: Chronic coxarthrosis, chronic lumbago.

Contra-indications: Acute lumbago, inflammation in the area of treatment.

Effects: Relaxes muscles, reduces spasms, stimulates blood circulation, calms, reduces pain.

Equipment: 1 wool blanket, 1 linen cloth, 1-2 meadow flower haypacks.

Procedure: Apply the haypack carefully on the client. Fasten haypack tightly and be careful not to burn the skin. In order to prevent heat from escaping, wrap the haypack snugly. The client can lie sideways or lie comfortably on the back. Leave on as long as the haypack feels warm to the client.

■

32

Some Important Procedures Adopted with Massage Therapy

Mud pack, genital bath, sponging, sunbath, fasting, deep breathing etc. are important procedures. Here I have described these procedure because one should know about these procedures along with Massage Therapy.

Mud Packs

The best way to prepare a mud pack is to take clay from about four inches below the surface of the earth. Ensure that the clay does not contain any impurities, like compost or pebbles. If there are any pebbles. grind the clay and pass it through a sieve. Mix it with cold water and see that it has a consistency like soft dough. It should stick and not be thin enough to slide down when used in the pack. If the pack is to be applied on the abdomen (from the navel to the pubes) spread the mud evenly on a piece of cloth. See that it is about half an inch thick. Then place it gently with the cloth up and the mud touching the skin. Remove the cloth and place a thick wollen piece of cloth on the mud. You may even let the cotton cloth remain over the mud, but cover it with a thick woollen. If that is done the patient can keep lying down without covering himself with a blanket or a sheet.

The mud pack should be used for 20 to 30 minutes. After it is removed, clean the skin using a soft piece of cloth dipped in cold water.

Clay is to be found in different shades in different places, but whatever the colour, it is equally beneficial. If the mud is loamy and has a tendency to stikc to the skin, some sand can be mixed with it.

Hip Bath

You must have seen specially made tubs for hip baths. The tub is oval in shape and one end of it is raised so that the patient can rest his back against it. This is the ideal tub for taking a hip bath.

Fill the tub with cold water. The level of the water should be so adjusted that it touches your navel when you sit in it. Your feet will be outside the tub and you can support them by keeping a low stool in front of the tub. You can rest your back against the raised portion of the tub and remain in that half supine position.

Take a rough towel and rub your abdomen from the right to the left. Do it gently so that the skin is not scraped. Do not apply too much pressure in rubbing.

A hip bath can be taken from ten to twenty minutes. Thin persons should take it for only ten minutes and the stout ones can continue for 20 minutes. During winter the duration of the hip bath should be reduced by about 25 per cent.

In the begining, the hip bath should be taken only for a minute or two; the time should be increased gradually to ten or twenty minutes, as indicated above.

If it is too cold, rub your body with your palms for five to seven minutes before getting into the tub. A vigorous rubbing of the body will bring warmth to it and you will not experience any discomfort when you start the hip bath.

Wipe your body with a towel when you get out of the tub, dress quickly and go for a walk or take some other exercise. Those too weak to engage in any such activity should get into bed and wrap a blanket around them and rest for half an hour to bring back warmth to their body.

You can take a bath a couple of hours after the hip bath and not before.

Genitals Bath

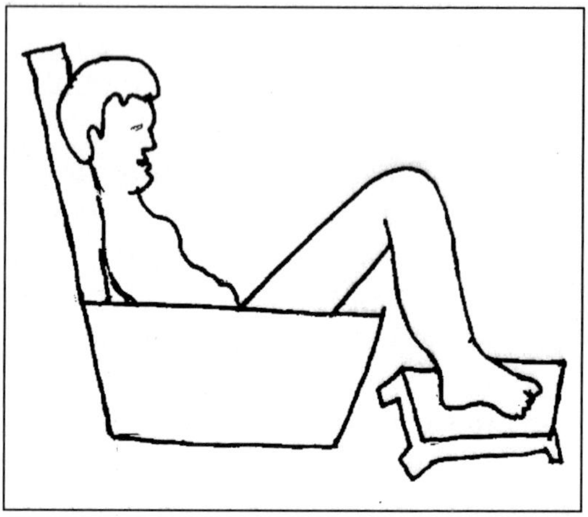

Genitals Bath

Keep a stool one foot long, six inches wide and six inches high in the tub. It would be all the better if there is a circular cut in front of it. If a stool is not readily available keep four bricks, two upon two to raise the level and sit on them. The water level in the tub should be such that it is one inch above the stool. The water should be cold; during summer the water of an earthen pitcher can be used for the purpose.

Take off your clothes and sit on the stool. Take a piece of cloth, dip it in water and gently rub your abdomen with it for two minutes. Then take hold of the foreskin of your penis in two fingers and rub it lightly with a soft piece of cloth dipping cold water often. This can be continued for ten to twenty minutes. A lean person can do it for only ten minutes, and the hefty one for as long as twenty minutes. After the rubbing of the foreskin is completed, rub the entire spine with a wet towel for two minutes. You can take hold of the wet towel in two hands and move it up and down on your spine.

Women should rub their abdomen. They should take a piece of soft cloth, pull up the lips of the vagina and rub them slowly. And in the end they should also rub the spine as above. No hip bath or genitals bath should be taken at the time of menstruation.

You must take exercise, walk or lie down in a bed and wrap yourself in a blanket to restore the body heat lost due to immersion in water.

If a tub is not available, this bath can be taken in the sum. In that case spread a wet towel on the stool on which you sit. Keep a bucket full of water near the stool and take the bath as indicated above.

How to Take a Bath

A bath is a daily ritual, but few people understand its purpose or importance. That is why most of us merely throw water over our heads and the bodies and think that we have done our duty. Throwing water over the body is beneficial but it is not what a bath is.

The twin purposes of a bath are: cleanliness and reactivating the circulation of the blood by the tingling sensation that cold water produces as it comes into contact with the skin. The first purpose, i.e. cleanliness, can be better served by hot water. The skin of the body has millions of pores through which the skin breathes as we do through our lungs. If the pores are clogged, the lungs are overworked. Overwork may lead to fatigue or exhaustion of the lungs. And then, closed pores do not pass any perspiration which the skin breathes as we do through our lungs. If the pores are clogged, the lungs are overworked.Overwork may lead to fatigue or exhaustion of the lungs. And then, closed pores do not pass any perspiration which is a must to clear the blood of morbid humours. Closed pores are a danger to the general health of human beings.

Cold water is also a cleansing agent, but it cannot deal with the grease and dirt infesting the pores of the skin. Hot water mixed with lemon juice is the best cleansing agent for the skin. Or, better still, take a lemon and roast it lightly over a fire. Then cut it into two parts, dip a part in hot water and rub it over your skin. This will cleanse your skin a s no soap can do. But a hot bath should not be taken daily. It generally brings lethargy, weakness and slows down the digestive processes. Once or twice a week is enough if you have to take a hot bath. The temperature of the water should not be more than one or two degree above body temperature.

A hot bath before retiring for the night is the best for your health. It helps you to sleep better and if you cover your body after a hot bath, it will save you from the danger of exposure. A bath, hot or cold should be taken one hour before meals or three hours after it.

Really hot water for a bath has its own advantages but it should be used sparingly. If you are suffereing from a cold, take a hot bath, cover yourself with woollens and get into bed. It will drive away the cold. A really hot bath when you are tired acts as a tonic: it drives away fatigue as nothing else does.

A bath with hot water has its used, but a daily bath should be with cold water. When the skin is cooled by the cold water, blood rushes to warm it up. The circulation of the blood is activated and the blood is also cleansed of many impurities. A slowed down circulation is a prelude to old age. A cold bath is, therefore, instrumental in keeping us young.

The best way to start a bath is to rub the whole of your body with your palms or with a rough towel. Start with your scalp , forehead, face and the neck . Then go on to your wrists and then to the shoulders through the arms. Afterwards rub your chest, the armpits and abdomen and the back. The feet should be the lst to receive attention. Keep your feet straight when you rub them. Start from the feet and come upto the thighs. In the begining, rub gently but later increase the pressure.

After the vigorous rubbing, take a cold bath. Wipe your body with a towel. Start with the head and then dry up the whole body. You will feel a peculiar kind of pleasure when you rub your body afte a bath. For weak persons a rubbing can do the job of exercise.

If this method of taking a bath is adopted, there will not be any danger of any skin eruptions or itch. The face will be free of pimples and other blemishes which mar its beauty. The skin will acquire a healthy glow and if it is rough and leathery, it will become pink and soft. You will have the feeling as if you had been having an oil massage.

If the palms of the hand are used to dry up the body after a bath instead of a towel, it will be doubly beneficial. It gives pleasant sensation during winter.

Wet Pack for the Waist

The bandage to be used as a wet pack for the waist should be seven to eight feet long and six inches broad. It should be of soft cotton cloth. Dip it in cold water, ring it lightly and wrap it around your waist. It should cover the area from the navel to a little above the pubes and should remain in direct contact with the skin. Cover the wet bandage with a woollen cloth of equal dimensions and secure with a safety pin or a string so that it does not loosen up.

There will be a cold sensation on the skin covered by the wet pack but after about ten minutes warmth will return. If you still feel cold after ten minutes, that is an indication that the bandage has been wrapped lightly and has to be tightend. Or, the bandage has not been properly wrung out or it is thicker than it should be.

The wet pack for the waist can be used from half an hour to two hours at a time.

Wet Pack for the Chest

The dimensions of the bandage for the chest should be the same as for the waist. It should be similarly dipped in cold water, wrung out and wrapped round the chest and covered by a woollen piece of cloth. It should be wrapped in such a way that it should cover the chest, the upper part of the shoulders and the corresponding portion of the back. The woollen covering for the wet pack should be secured with a safety pin or a piece of string as in the case of the waist pack.

This pack can also be used for half an hour to two hours.

Sun Bath

Sun bath is an important tool of the naturopath. Even though people in the west use it for cosmetic purposes, it plays an important part in restoring health.

In Indian conditions, the ideal times for a sun bath during summer is six to six thirty in the morning and during winter from seven to seven thirty.

Take off all your clothes and sit in a secluded corner away from interruptions. The whole of your body should be exposed to the health-giving rays of the sun.

In the beginning take a sun bath for only two to three minutes but increase the timing gradual to fefteen to twenty minutes.

When the sunlight is very hot, cover your head with a towel. If you cannot find a secluded place to take the sun bath, cover yourself with a light cotton sheet.

Sun-bath for Inducing Perspiration

Sweat can be induced through a sun bath. For this purpose the sun is hot enough at ten to eleven in the morning in summer and two to three in the afternoon in winter. Take hot water and lie down naked on a mattress or blanket spread on the floor. If the wind is strong, chose a place in the lee of the wind.

You will start sweating in about ten to fifteen minutes after you have lied down. After fifteen to twenty minutes. Whether you sweat or not, you must take a cold bath just after it.

Some people may not perspire in the begining but after repeating the sun bath for three of four days, their sweat glands will be activated and they will perspire.

You must cover you head with a wet towel while taking a sun bath, but at the same time go on sipping warm water to aid the body to produce the sweat.

Sponging the Body

When you are running a temperature, a sponge bath is more advisable than a bath. The patient should be covered with a sheet or blanket and his body should be wiped with a wet towel. Wipe his feet first, one after the other. Rub them with the wet towel for four to five minutes and then wipe them with a dry towel. But even when the feet have been dried rub them with the palms of the hand so that some heat is generated in the body. In the case of fever, such rubbing is not advised.

After the feet have been attended to go to the calves and the rest of the legs, the abdomen, the chest, the back, the face and the neck. The hands should be rubbed for five to six minutes and the abdomen, chest and the back a little longer.

The total time taken for a sponge bath is on an average half an hour. The ideal time for a sponge bath is mid day.

Fasting

Nothing but water should be taken when you are fasting. The intake of water must be two to two and a half litres. One feels fresh if one continues drinking water and the intake of water also helps the expulsion of morbid matter from the body.

In the evening of the first day of the fast and the morning after, an enema of hot water should be taken to clean the bowels.

One day's fasting should be followed by a food intake 25 percent less than one normally takes. A two days fast should be followed by ingestion of fruits only the next day; normal food should follow the next day. A three day's fast should be followed the next day by fruit juices and soup of vegetables (the soup must be clear, without addition of any thickening agents or condiments). On the fifth day eat fruits only and on the sixth breakfast on fruits, lunch on bread and boiled vegetables and repeat a fruit diet for your dinner. It is only after wards that you should resume your normal diet.

Fruits, Fruit Juices and Milk Diets

When you have been advised to live on fruit juices or juices or soups of vegetables, you should take sbout 250 millilitres of fruit juice or juice or clear soup of a vegetable three to four times in the day. The best juices are those of oranges pineapple, rose apple, raspberry and tomatoes. If the juice is too thick, mix it with plain water in the proportion of 1:¾th.

Juice of gourd, tomatoes and carrot can be taken in its natural form. If you do not have a juicer (a machine to extract the juice of fruits) grate the fruits or vegetables and sqeeze then through fine muslin or other fine meshed cloth.

Other vegetables have to be half a kilogramme and should be boiled in 250 millilitres of water and the juice drunk.

When you are living on fruit, take them thrice daily. But take one kind of fruit at one meal. For example, you can take tomatoes for breakfast, oranges at lunch time and apples for your dinner. If you can take the same fruit at all meal times, it would be still better.

The total intake of fruits in the day should not be more than one to one and a half kilogrammes.

When a diet of fruit and milk is indicated, take 250 to 300 millilitres of milk with the fruits. If your appetite improves, as it should the quantity of the milk can be increased to half a litre at one time. Unboiled milk should be taken in the morning and even during lunch time milk boiled in the morning can be ingested. Sip the milk as you munch the fruit. It will be more beneficial than eating the fruit and drinking the milk.

Even when you are on a diet of fruit juices, do not forget to drink one to two litres of water in the day. If your bowels do not move automatically during the fruit and milk diet, take recourse to an enema. But the bowels must be evacuated properly and no morbid humours or substances should be allowed to accumulate in the body.

Intake of Water

One must drink one to one and a half litres of water in 24 hours. The best time for taking water is the first thing in the morning, one hour before meals and two hours after. If you must drink water during the meals, see that the quantity does not exceed 200 to 250 millilitres. If you have taken water one hour before the meals, you will not feel the need to take it during eating. But still, water may be taken during the meal according to need and inclination.

Walking, Deep Breathing and Sleep

During a walk, you must move briskby. Your back should be straight and the arms moving.

The normal speed of walking should be about four miles per hour. Take a different route for a walk every day as that would be more enjoyable instead of taking the same route every day.

Five to six miles walk in the morning and two to three miles in the evening is the best. Those who are starting to take a walk should not overstrain themselves but increases the distance gradually.

Deep breathing

Deep breaths should be taken during a walk. Inhalation should become a natural rhythm with you. Inhalation andexhalation should not be done slowly.

Sleep

Sleep should be sufficient to give a sense of relief from exhaustion. But do not oversleep, nor laze about in bed when you are not sleeping. The ideal time for sleep is from nine o'clock in the night to five in the morning. Those who feel sleepy all the time return to normal sleeping hours after some days.

During summer, a siesta for an hour or so will refresh you. If you cannot sleep, relax for an hour after lunch.

Inhalation and Vaporisation

Inhalations are considered to be highly effective, as the olfactory (smelling) receptors have direct links with the brain. Inhalations are said to quite useful and effective in routing skin-care treatment, respiratory conditions, such as colds, coughs, sore throats, catarrh, blocked nasal passages but use with utmost care if you are an asthmatic, Vaporisers and scented baths can also prove relaxing and invigorating, depending on the oil chosen for a specific physical/mental problems

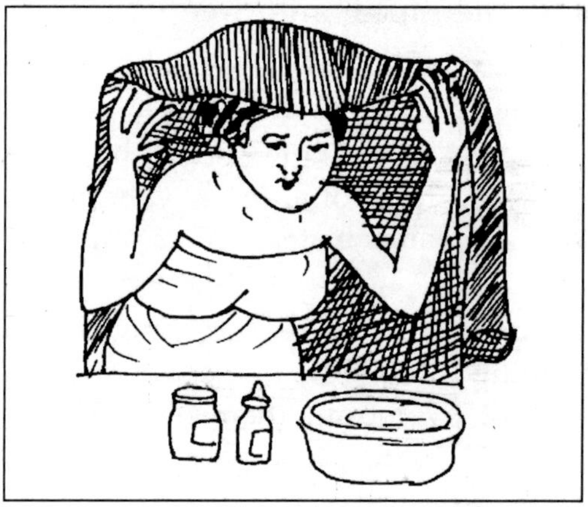

Vaporisation and Inhalation

For inhalations add 4 drops of a suitable essential oil to a bowl of steaming water and then lean over the bowl with you head covered by a towel but keep your eyes closed . Breathe in deeply. Initially, inhalation may be a bit problematic but once the blocked and stuck up nostritls are cleared of trapped muslces, inhalation will automatically improve.

You can use eucalyptus or peppermint oil (4–6 drops or either or 2–3 drops of each of the oils). If steam inhalation is not feasible, you can put 4-5 drops of the oil on a hanky (tissue cloth) hold it to your nose and take deep breathes. But do not inhale directly from the bottle itself.

■ ■ ■

Other Books on
HEALTH

1. Yoga for Health and Relaxation **(New)**
2. Yoga for All **(New)**
3. Yoga for Daily Life **(New)**
4. Complete Book of Yoga **(New)**
5. Yoga Therapy **(New)**
6. A Guide to Your Pregnancy **(New)**
7. Ayurveda for All
8. A Guide to Migraine, Airthritis, Cervical Spondylosis, and Backache
9. Body and Beauty Care
10. Child Care and Nutrition
11. Naturopathy Modern Way of Life
12. First Aid How to Handle an Accident
13. Acupressure in Daily Life
14. Look Younger at Any Age
15. HIV/AIDS - Transmission, Prevention and A. Therapies
16. Diabetics and Diet
17. Increase your Height & Loose your Weight
18. Make Fitness A Way of Life
19. Common Problems of Children
20. Handbook of Nutrition & Dietetics
21. A Guide to Massage Therapy
22. A Guide to Family Medicine
23. A Guide to Digestive Disorders
24. Complete Book of Child Care
25. A Guide to Homoeopathy
26. Life Begins at 40
27. Alternative Therapies

28. How to Overcome Stress
29. Obesity
30. Self Motivation
31. Women Disorders and Pregnancy
32. A Guide to Body Pains
33. Sex Education
34. Common Diseases and Cure
35. Pranayama for Better Life
36. Herbal Home Remedies
37. A Guide to Beauty & Skin Care
38. A Guide to Heart Care
39. A Guide to High Blood Pressure
40. Cancer Causes and Prevention
41. Nature Cure for Common Diseases
42. Good Health Through Food and Regimen
43. A Guide to Allergies
44. A Guide to Aging
45. Ayurveda for Health & Beauty

Lotus PRESS

Unit No. 220, 2nd Floor, 4735/22, Prakash Deep Building,
Ansari Road, Darya Ganj, New Delhi- 110002
• E-mail : lotuspress1984@gmail.com, www.lotuspress.co.in